AN INTRODUCTION TO
MASSAGE

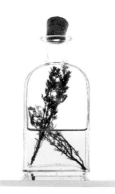

AN INTRODUCTION TO
MASSAGE

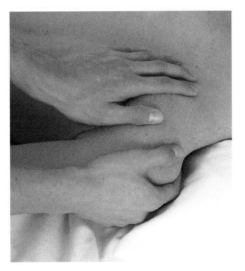

SUSAN MUMFORD

LONDON   NEW YORK   SYDNEY   TORONTO

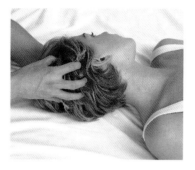
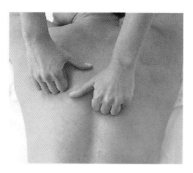
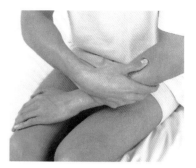

Photography by Richard Truscott

Commissioning Editor Sian Facer
Executive Art Editor Keith Martin
Art Editor Trinity Fry
Art Director Jacqui Small
Editor Linda Gibson

This edition published 1995 by BCA by arrangement with
Hamlyn, an imprint of Reed Consumer Books Limited

CN 8154

Printed in Spain by Cayfosa, Barcelona

Note: Massage should not be considered as a replacement for professional medical
treatment; a physician should be consulted in all matters relating to health and
especially in relation to any symptoms which may require diagnosis or medical
attention. Care should be taken during pregnancy, particularly in the use of
essential oils. Essential oils should not be ingested and should be used
for babies and children only on professional advice.

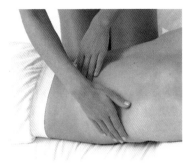
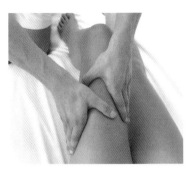
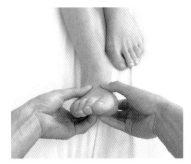

CONTENTS

INTRODUCTION

I have always thought that the beauty of massage lies in it being such a simple, direct form of human contact – there is nothing to hide behind, no instruments or machines, only you and your partner. Massage holds such a fascination because it fulfills a basic need, satisfying the desire both to touch and be touched. It can also be used in so many different ways. Having acquired some basic massage skills, you will find yourself forever popular at parties, work, or on the beach. It is fun to be able to just sit down anywhere and give a five minute neck or shoulder rub, and then for you both to run off and do something else.

In another sense, there can be nothing so deeply rewarding as creating an intimate massage space for a friend. With the same set of skills, you can provide genuine release from long-term tension, backache or a dip in confidence. Watch the light creep back behind your partner's smile as he or she visibly unravels in front of you! With friends, family and lovers, massage can provide the framework to strengthen your contact and knowledge of each other. If you want to take massage further, and this is certainly where my own interest lies, it can be a very special way of becoming more aware of the deeper levels on which our energies connect and interact with each other.

Massage is a basic, fundamental skill that all of us should have. While it requires learning some basic techniques and strokes, perhaps the most important ingredient is the individuality both of you bring to the experience. At the same time, sensitivity, generosity, warmth and openness are all essential for a massage to mean more than just a series of movements. In fact, an inspired massage is an opportunity for two people to be able to go beyond themselves, nourish the spirit and release creativity. For something that is so simple, massage has profound and far-reaching effects.

This book is intended to be used as a comprehensive guide to giving a basic massage. It will take you right through from the very beginning to being able to give a full body massage. The massage is presented in stages, so that you can learn about massage preparation and the techniques you will need before combining them in a massage. People often find the idea of being able to massage appealing, and simply need some encouragement to take that first step! I recommend trying the massage first of all with a friend you feel comfortable with. Then if you approach it with a sense of exploration, as well as humor, your discoveries, successes, and even mistakes, can develop and grow into your own personal style.

How to use the book

An introduction to the way the massage progresses through the book may be helpful here. As there is nothing to beat hands-on instruction when you are learning, the massage itself has been presented as closely as possible to how you would actually be taught. You would naturally learn in steps, and certainly not learn everything at once. So, the massage has been divided into easy stages in which you will have the opportunity to complete and practice one stage before going on to the next. The sections build upon the information you have just learnt. While you may want to follow each step at first, the idea is for you to develop a collection of strokes from which you can then create your own massage.

Before Beginning is a guide to the basics of anatomy and physiology. This helps to give a clear visual idea of exactly where you will be placing your hands. It cannot, however, be stressed enough that all this is intended as background information, and that a theoretical approach to massage is always more of a hindrance than a help!

Getting Started, contains a guide to oils and aromatherapy essences you can use to enhance the massage, and it includes simple recipes you can try. Some introductory exercises are then included so that you can become more familiar with your own body before beginning to work on someone else, noticing your flexibility and limitations. This will help when you come to massage your partner.

The massage strokes are approached gradually by trying them out on yourself first to find out what feels good. It also gives some ideas for you to increase the sensitivity of your hands.

Simple Techniques demonstrates the strokes you will be using during the body massage. Each technique is shown on several parts of the body to give a better all-round idea of how they can be used. It is best to try these out before you begin the massage.

Simple Massage flows on from this and contains a step-by-step guide to a basic massage, incorporating the techniques just shown. Follow each step to begin with, and you can then go on to develop your own favourite strokes and style. Do not, however, in any way feel that you need to stop right here. The techniques and sequence you have learned are more than sufficient to enable you to give a thoroughly satisfying body massage. However, they may also serve as your introduction to the world of massage and whet your appetite for more! Feel free to use the massage as a foundation for adding new techniques that you may either go on to learn or invent. There are so many avenues to explore, and however much you learn, the more you will find there is to discover.

Finally, just as important as starting a massage is the way it ends. After Massage concentrates on making sure you both get the most from it, take time to relax afterwards, and, very importantly, put back what you have given out.

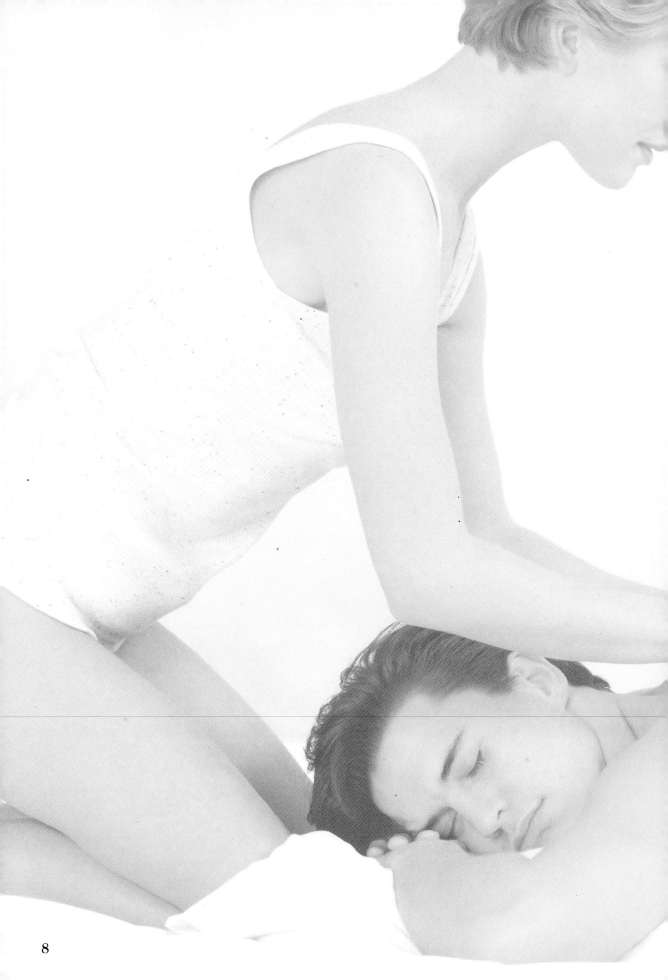

BEFORE BEGINNING

Being at the beginning of something new is always exciting. However, it can appear daunting when you are faced with something large and unknown without really knowing where to begin. Hopefully, by approaching massage in manageable stages, actually beginning will be much easier! The temptation is to want to massage right away, but before going on to the practical aspects, familiarize yourself with this opening section. Having an idea of what you are working with, what you will need to start, and why you should massage in the first place all help to give confidence and meaning to what you do. Massage has so many connotations. For whatever reason you decide to massage, the practice has real value and proven results.

INTRODUCTION TO MASSAGE

What is massage?

Massage is a form of structured touch. The hands, or sometimes other parts of the body, such as the forearms or elbows, are used to glide over the skin and apply pressure to the underlying muscles in a series of movements that involve variously stroking, rubbing, kneading and pressing. It can be either soothing or stimulating, and when used in conjunction with a focus on energy, can affect the body, mind, spirit and emotions. Massage is an ancient, revered art that has been practiced for centuries. The ancient Egyptians, Greeks, and Romans all used massage for healing and health, as well as pleasure. In India, China and Japan, massage forms an integral part of whole systems of medicine, while reference to massage in China dates back from between two to three thousand years B.C.

What does massage do?

Massage does not actually do anything to the body! However, what it does is to stimulate and encourage the body to carry out its normal functions. In other words, massage is not something you do to another person, it is a process that you initiate, to which the body then responds. Massage provides the stimulation, and the body does the work.

The therapeutic benefits produced by massage include loosening of muscular tension, toning and firming the muscles, and stimulating the circulation of the blood and lymph. Through too much or not enough exercise, or physical or mental tension, the waste products from muscular activity (carbon dioxide, lactic acid and urea), can accumulate in the muscles, preventing the fibres from sliding easily over each other and producing an increase in muscle tone. Massage aids drainage of these wastes, principally lactic acid, freeing the muscles and restoring normal function. It also reminds the muscles how

it feels to be relaxed. Massage helps stimulate lymph drainage and the circulation of the blood. This will improve the appearance of the skin, which is the largest organ of the body. Healthy skin has a positive mental effect, and many skin problems are stress-related. The state of one's skin often reflects one's general inner state.

Massage affects the nerves as well as the muscles, acting on the autonomic nervous system to produce a general feeling of relaxation. The stimulation of sensory nerve endings in the skin is relayed to the brain via the central nervous system contributing to the feel-good factor. This then has an effect on the rest of the body, and will help reduce the effects of stress. The nervous system also controls the vascular system. A lack of vascular supply results in decreased efficiency in drainage and supply of blood. The relaxation process helps produce a more natural abdominal breathing pattern, which is vital to the function of the abdominal organs. Stress and fatigue, caused by the accumulation of waste products, can be reduced, and the metabolic process made more effective.

Massage works on the muscles, and can affect the fibrous tissue surrounding the joints, but any skeletal problems will need to be dealt with separately. It is certainly not a cure–all, but can help enormously through relaxation, helping the body restore its natural balance. It is unfortunate that many people will only discover massage once they develop a problem. It is, in fact, an excellent preventative. And, yes, it does feels great!

Who can benefit?

Massage is for everyone, absolutely. Anyone can massage. It is true that some people have a better natural touch than others, but there is no reason why everyone cannot learn. And anyone can be massaged. There are certain contraindications, but in general everyone can benefit regardless of their age or physical ability. All of us need touch. It is one of our earliest life experiences and needs.

Research has shown how a lack of touch can restrict normal development in babies. Experiments on baby monkeys showed how they preferred a soft, surrogate-mother figure made of cloth which they could snuggle up to, rather than a harshly constructed wire one which could supply them with food. Babies in incubators who are touched and stroked fare better, so do hospital patients who are touched and reassured. Even people borrowing books from the library experienced a positive effect when the librarian lightly touched them on the hand.

Touch makes us feel wanted. Without touch we become withdrawn. This is the reason why massage can particularly help people suffering bereavement or loss, or those not in a physical relationship. Touch is a means of communication, affirmation and expression, providing a sense of identity and helping to build confidence and self-esteem. (It does not have to be only with humans, animals can provide a wonderful sense of touch and companionship, but everyone needs to have something!) In an increasingly over-stimulated and desensitized world, where mental activity has superseded the physical, massage provides the opportunity to keep in touch with your body and to feel it fully. The all-over glow of being comfortable with your skin is something we often miss out on.

Following a massage, many people will experience the sense of being a connected whole as opposed to a disconnected series of parts. They are also more aware of their physical boundaries and experience the sense of their feet being more firmly planted on the ground. Massage provides that vital and essential sense of touch, of being looked after, without the pressure of having to give back anything in return.

Massage provides balance, especially if the person giving the massage is concentrating and using their energy effectively. If you are feeling over-stimulated, massage can help sedate and calm, or if you are feeling sluggish, it can help wake you up. It can also be used to help specific problems, such as back and shoulder aches, period pains, coughs, headaches and so on, and can be used as part of the process of recuperation after injury or illness. However, be very clear that you are not aiming to cure, and that long-term or acute problems need a check-up and professional help. Massage can be used before and after sport or exercise, to help the body warm up, or to relax and tone the muscles afterwards, preventing stiffness the next day. By helping tone the muscles, massage can help as part of a fitness or beauty programme, while the use of oils combined with massage will help stimulate cell renewal and improve the elasticity of the skin. Some people worry about their bodies, thinking they are too fat or unattractive to be massaged. However, in my experience, massage can have the opposite effect, and make you feel much better about your body.

Tension accounts for a lot more problems than we perhaps realize. Most people nowadays are suffering from one form of stress-related condition or another. This can be felt as physical tension, resulting in tight, knotted muscles, or mental overactivity and anxiety, which will then affect the body function. For anyone who is suffering from stress, massage can help reduce the physical effects of tension, and calm the mind and emotions, while restoring vital energy. The touch and attention of massage helps deal with stress.

The connection between mind and body is such that being in good shape, physically, affects the mind, and being mentally relaxed helps your body to function better.

ANATOMY GUIDE

The muscles

Skeletal muscles provide the shape of the body. These are voluntary muscles under conscious control, such as the arms and legs, as opposed to involuntary muscles, which include those of the heart and digestive system. Each muscle consists of bundles of elastic muscle fibers, each surrounded by cell membrane, bound together by a connective sheath. This is known as the muscle belly. The muscles are primarily attached to the bones at either end by highly resistant connective tissue, or tendons. The points at which the muscles attach to the bone are known as the origin (the bone the muscle does not move), and the insertion (the bone the muscle does move when it contracts). In normal body function the muscles work in pairs or groups, contracting and relaxing in order to propel the body. Responding to signals from the

A guide to the superficial muscles

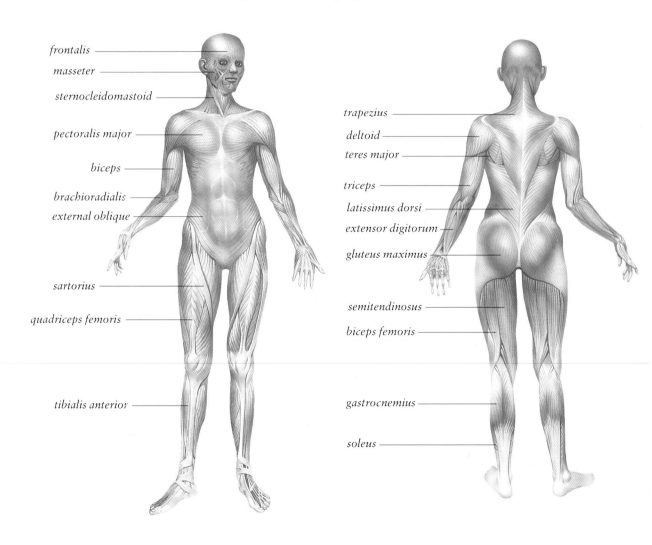

frontalis
masseter
sternocleidomastoid
pectoralis major
biceps
brachioradialis
external oblique
sartorius
quadriceps femoris
tibialis anterior

trapezius
deltoid
teres major
triceps
latissimus dorsi
extensor digitorum
gluteus maximus
semitendinosus
biceps femoris
gastrocnemius
soleus

brain, a muscle will contract. As it does so the fibers slide toward each other, shortening both the length and width of the muscle. This causes movement. The muscle that contracts is called the synergist. The muscles which relax during the same movement are called antagonists. The synergist and antagonist will change depending on the particular movement. When the muscles remain in a contracted state this is known as an increase in resting tone. To function, the muscles need blood containing large amounts of glucose and oxygen and produce, as by-products, the waste materials of carbon dioxide, lactic acid and urea, which are carried away by the venous system and lymph. Where there is a shortening of muscle function, some of this waste may remain in the muscles, causing stiffness, and preventing the fibers from easily sliding over each other.

A guide to the major organs of the body

THE LUNGS
The lungs are spongy structures, protected by the ribs, into which air is drawn. Through the lungs, oxygen enters the bloodstream and carbon dioxide is expired.

THE KIDNEYS
The kidneys are concerned with the filtering of waste products, and the absorption of water, glucose, protein and vitamins. Their function is to conserve water within the body, and return it to the tissues, the remainder passing through the body as urine.

THE HEART
The heart is a muscle. It acts like a pump, contracting to circulate oxygenated blood around the body, and return deoxygenated blood to the lungs.

THE STOMACH
The stomach stores and digests food, breaking it down by means of enzymes in preparation for processing in the small intestine.

THE LIVER
The function of the liver is to absorb nutrients from the blood, to break down fats, carbohydrates and proteins, store vitamins, and detoxify the blood. It is also concerned with the production of bile.

THE LARGE INTESTINE
The large intestine is concerned with the absorption of water, vitamins and minerals, which pass to the liver. The waste products pass through the body.

THE SMALL INTESTINE
The small intestine further breaks down food by means of enzymes and digests sugars, fats and proteins. The majority of nutrients are absorbed here.

The skeleton

The skeleton is made up of some 206 bones, and provides the support and framework for the body. The bones themselves are made up of living tissue, comprising fibers, cells, and mineral salts, and are long, short, flat, irregular or sesamoid (formed in tendons). Each bone is covered by a thick layer of fibrous tissue which has an abundant blood supply, with cell-producing marrow in both the central shaft and spongy layer at either end, which is then capped by cartilage. The bones provide protection for vital organs, such as the brain and heart, and allow the body to move through their connection at the joints. They also provide sites of attachment for the muscles. The axial skeleton is the main structure including the skull, spine, and ribs. The appendicular skeleton provides the supporting framework for the arms and legs, includes the pectoral and pelvic girdles and moves more freely. The vertebrae of the spine are divided into the seven cervical, supporting the neck and skull (the seventh is the bony prominence just below the base of the neck); the 12 thoracic, to which the ribs are attached; the five lumbar, providing the main support for the body; the five sacral, which are fused together to form the sacrum, distributing the weight of the body to the hips; and the four coccygeal, fused together to form the coccyx.

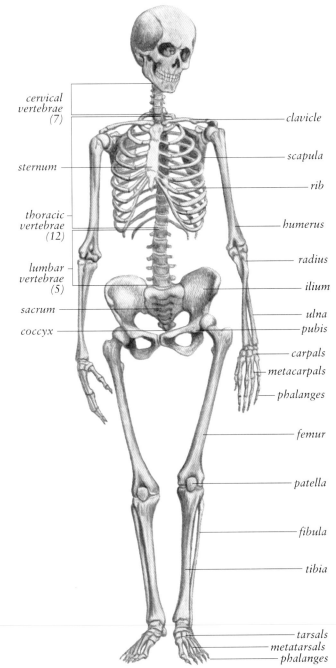

Joints

The point at which two bones connect is a joint. The most common is a synovial joint. Here the bones connect within a cavity surrounded by a fluid-secreting membrane, which protects the cartilage and reduces friction during movement. It is contained by a fibrous capsule and supported by tendons and ligaments. The ball-and-socket type, found at the shoulder and hip, permits a wide range of movement. Here the round head of one bone fits into the socket shape of the other. Hinge joints are found at the elbow and knee. The bone surfaces swing about each other permitting a more limited movement.

The ball-and-socket shoulder joint

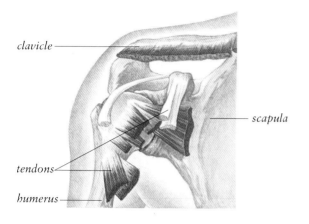

clavicle

scapula

tendons

humerus

The hinge knee joint

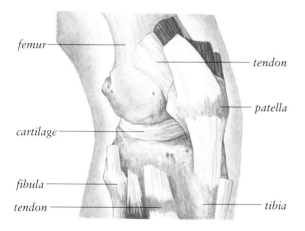

femur

tendon

patella

cartilage

fibula

tendon

tibia

The nervous system

The nervous system consists of the central nervous system (the brain and spinal cord), and the peripheral nervous system (the cranial and spinal nerves branching out to all areas of the body). In response to stimuli, sensory receptors in the skin, soft tissue and muscles send impulses via sensory nerves to the central nervous system. Responding to signals from the brain, motor nerves send impulses to the muscles resulting in movement and activity. The autonomic nervous system is concerned with the involuntary movements of the organs, blood vessels and glands. It divides into the sympathetic nervous system, which governs involuntary responses such as increased heartbeat, respiration and sweat, and the parasympathetic nervous system, which is concerned with a reduction in activity, and processes such as digestion and rest. These systems work together to maintain balanced body function.

Circulation of the blood

The cardiovascular system consists of the heart, arteries carrying oxygenated blood from the heart, veins returning deoxygenated blood, and capillaries supplying nutrients to the tissues and removing wastes. The blood comprises plasma, red cells supplying oxygen from the lungs to the tissues and cells and removing carbon dioxide, white cells, important to the immune system fighting bacteria and secreting antibodies, and platelets, responsible for clotting. The heart, acting like a pump, has four chambers, two dealing with circulation through the lungs, two with circulation to the rest of the body. Blood in the arteries is pumped at high pressure, the veins operating at lower pressure. In the legs blood flow is assisted by muscle contraction and valves to return blood supply to the heart. The lymph system, arising from the vascular system, helps drain tissues and return fluid to the heart. The lymph flows through its own vessel system, draining into ducts. Nodes or glands filter the fluid, producing lymphocites to neutralize bacteria. Flow is aided by muscle contraction.

PREPARATION FOR MASSAGE

Where to massage.

In theory, you can massage anywhere. It all depends on the type of massage you are giving. If you are adapting your massage for a quick neck and shoulder or hand massage, for example, you can simply do it wherever you happen to be. However, do follow the basic principles so that your partner is sitting with a supported back, either on the floor or on a chair, and make sure they do not slouch by supporting the forehead or chest with your hand if necessary. You can then massage outdoors, in the office or wherever. It is equally important that you massage from a comfortable position, without having to twist or strain. If, however, you are giving a full body massage, you need to choose your location a little more carefully. You will need to find a place where there is enough room for your partner to lie flat and for you to be able to move around them, and somewhere preferably that is quiet, comfortable and warm, where you will not be disturbed. A living room or bedroom floor is fine. However, the massage surface needs to be firm enough so that your partner will be supported and not sink into it, so do not massage on the bed as this is far too soft. If you are planning to do a lot of massage, then it is worth investing in a massage table. This is less intimate, but will also be less of a strain on your back.

The importance of your posture cannot be overemphasized. As well as avoiding a strain on your muscles, keeping the spine relaxed but straight as you perform the movements will significantly enhance your massage. It is also worth mentioning that as you are the person giving the massage, you need to be in a place where you feel comfortable. If you are happier in your own home, where you will have your things to hand, know what kind of coming and going there will be, and can keep an eye on the time, then ask your partner to travel to you.

The best time to massage

Again, this depends on the massage. The best time is ideally when you are feeling fresh and enthusiastic. Some people prefer to give or have a massage in the morning, others prefer later in the day. A neck and shoulder massage can be done at almost any time, on the spot if you are happy to do it. A body massage can be almost as flexible, taking certain points into consideration. Avoid massaging after a heavy meal. This applies especially to your partner, as the system is busy digesting food, and the pressure can feel uncomfortable. In the same way, do not drink alcohol before or immediately after a massage. Drinking before a massage dulls its effect, speeds up the absorption process and can make you feel sick. Directly after a massage also has a negative effect, and the alcohol will affect you much more quickly. (Massage can actually help with the effects of a mild hangover by helping to clear the system. However, if it is severe, the body will be far too sensitive.)

You should plan your massage when both of you have free time and do not have to rush. This means setting aside at least 90 minutes (up to an hour for a longer massage and a good 15 minutes either side). You also need to take into account the effects that massage has. If your partner has to go to work, a deep relaxation massage would be unsuitable. Some people do indeed like to have a massage before work or in a lunchbreak, to relax before an important performance or to get in shape before a run. This is fine as long as you adapt your massage to more stimulating strokes. It is also important you know this beforehand. As always, you must take your own needs into account. Do not massage late at night, as this will be too stimulating. While massage can help transform your state of mind, if you are preoccupied, busy, tired, or in a bad mood, this is not the time for you to give out any more of your energy.

What you will need

In order for the massage to go smoothly, have everything laid out beforehand. You will need a comfortable but firm surface for your partner to lie on, so start with a foam mat or small futon, for example, on the floor. You could even use a folded duvet or sleeping bag. You will then need a sheet to cover your surface, towels to cover your partner, pillows or cushions for the head or legs, and possibly a cushion for you to kneel on. You will need the oil at room temperature, extra heating available if necessary, soft lighting, some tissues to wipe off excess oil, and somewhere to wash your hands. If you have an answer machine, remember to switch it on. It is also a good idea to have a clock, and set a time limit before you start. When you begin to massage, especially, you can easily run over time, which is tiring for you, and your partner may be wondering when the massage is going to end! Add your own personal touches to make your massage room inviting, such as flowers, an aromatherapy burner, or music. These may seem like small points, but attention to detail makes all the difference, and means you can both put all your concentration into the massage.

Before you start

Before you begin to massage, agree a time limit with your partner, and make sure you know if they have to go to work afterwards, or, for example, do not want oil near their hair or face. Next, you need to ask a few questions before the massage begins. Check your partner's health, and make sure you know about any current illnesses, medication, or on-going problems such as neck or shoulder tension. Find out if there are particular parts of the body they would like massaged, or if there are any areas you should avoid. Even if you know your partner well, do not miss this stage out.

Contraindications

This means the circumstances in which you need to be careful, or should not massage at all. In general, as long as you are sensitive, you will not do any harm.

PREGNANCY: Massage during pregnancy can feel wonderful. However, at all stages of pregnancy, you should only work gently. Avoid massaging over the abdomen during the first four months, simply rest your hands instead, and thereafter circle very lightly. Check the list of essential oils carefully. Depending on the stage of pregnancy, you will need to adapt your partner's massage position.

INJURIES: Do not massage directly over recent scar tissue, injuries, sprains, open cuts or wounds. These will heal by themselves. However, gentle massage around the injury can be helpful.

ILLNESSES: Do not massage directly over a tumor, skin rash, or massage if your partner has a heart condition. Massage can actually be very good for the heart, but seek professional advice first. If in doubt, always consult your doctor or a health professional beforehand.

VARICOSE VEINS: Do not massage over varicose veins, but simply brush your hands over the leg lightly instead.

PAINS: Be practical. Never try to cure. If your partner has persistent aches, pains, muscular or spinal problems, or experiences any sharp pain during massage, consult your doctor.

Finally, to make sure your movements feel smooth, remove your jewellry (your partner should do the same), and make sure you have filed nails. Strong perfume can also interfere with your partner's enjoyment. Always wash your hands before and after each massage.

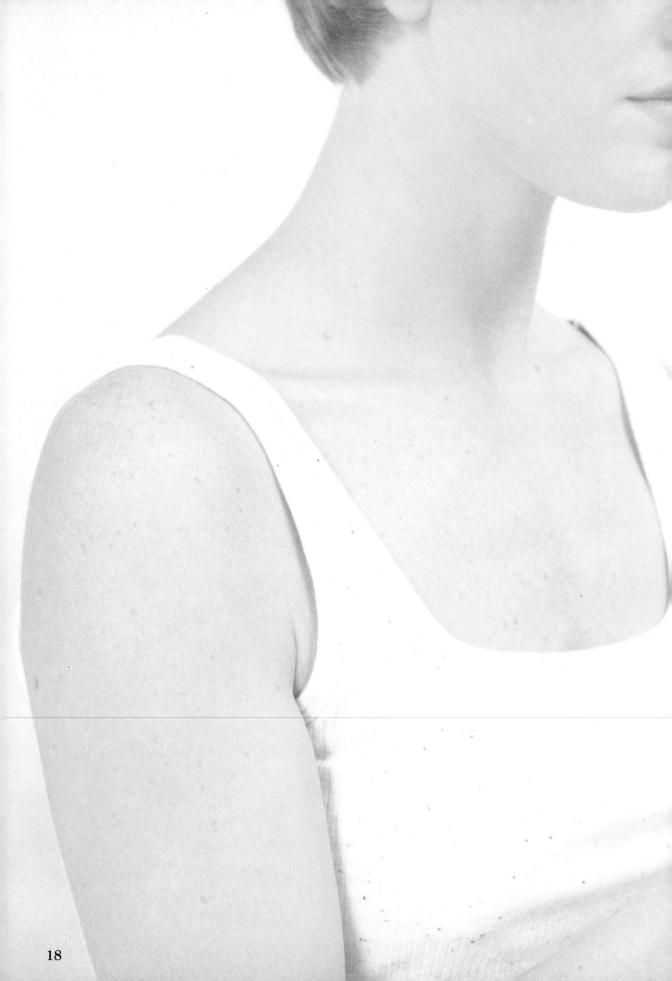

GETTING STARTED

A good massage needs a little careful thought and preparation. The amount of effort you put in will never be lost. The use of oils is exhilarating, but again you need some background information before you start. First get a feel for the oils, then you can begin to experiment. Similarly, trying out the strokes on yourself, and finding out more about your own body are an inevitable part of the massage process. The more you know about yourself, and the more attention you pay to developing the feeling in your hands, the more successful your massages will be. Not only do you learn more, but your partner will feel your enthusiasm, and directly benefit from all your time and effort.

OILS

Part of the preparation for massage is the selection and use of oils. The purpose of using oil is to help your hands move over your partner's body without pulling or stretching the skin. Most people like the feel of oil, although you do not absolutely have to use it. Some use talcum powder, and some strokes can be done through the clothes. However, if you choose to use oils, it is a good idea to have a selection prepared before you start.

The basic oil is called a base or carrier oil, and this is generally a vegetable or nut oil. You can use mineral oil, but this is not easily absorbed by the skin. The most popular carrier oils are grapeseed or sweet almond. Personally, I find almond oil is a little too cloying, and prefer grapeseed with about five or ten per cent almond oil added. Carrot, apricot or peach kernel, avocado, wheat germ and jojoba oils, which are much richer, can also be used. They are not recommended over large areas, but are excellent mixed in with other oils. A teaspoonful of wheatgerm oil can be used as an antioxidant to preserve your mixtures.

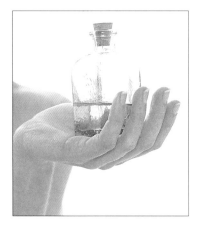

These oils can then be used as carriers for essential oils. This means that they can be used to dissolve the essential oils, helping them penetrate the skin. (This takes around thirty minutes.) Again you do not need to use the essences, but they are delightful and enhance the massage. Essential oils are the essences of plants that are extracted principally by means of steam distillation. Each oil contains the life force, quality and personality of the plant in concentrated form. The oil is produced by glands within the plant, be it in the leaves, roots or flowers, and it is this essence that is extracted. The oils are highly concentrated and potent, and should never be used directly on the skin as they will cause irritation. In too high a concentration they may have their opposite effect. Each oil has a rate of volatility, or rate at which it will evaporate, and these categories are divided into top, middle and base notes. The top notes have a high rate of volatility, and a higher vibration. They tend to have an immediate effect on the mind, and are generally quickening and uplifting. Middle notes are used to help the organs and functions of the body, while the base notes are sedative in effect, and can be used to anchor the top notes in a mixture. Essential oils can be used separately, but when mixed they interact with each other, enhancing and changing the quality of the whole. You usually use between two and four oils in any mixture; when using four have at least one middle note. While aromatherapy is an art in itself, essential oils can successfully be used to create certain moods, to stimulate or relax, and as long as you are not relying on tham as cures in any sense, can be used to help with minor ailments, such as blocked sinuses, skin irritations and aching muscles.

The use of oils is very personal. They affect us through their odor, as well as being absorbed through the skin. Smell is one of the most primitive brain functions, and one of the most evocative. Therefore, in mixing oils, preference plays a great part and is very much a matter of what feels right. If you or your partner do not like a smell, there is no point in using it. Similarly, as you massage you will naturally absorb oil through your hands, so if an oil affects you adversely, you should simply not use it. Use the oils sparingly, with just enough for your hands and the amount your partner's skin can absorb.

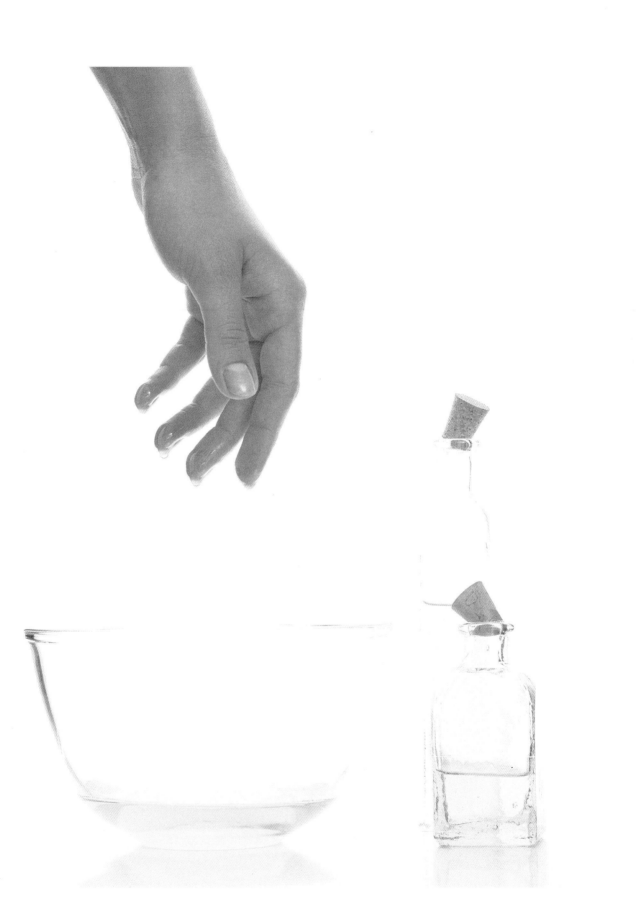

A GUIDE TO SOME COMMON OILS & THEIR PROPERTIES

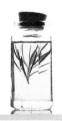

BASE OILS

GRAPESEED
A light, inexpensive carrier oil. Excellent for general use. Can be used on its own, or as the base for a mixture.

SWEET ALMOND
Another popular and widely used carrier oil. It can be used on its own, or as the base for a mixture.

APRICOT OR PEACH KERNEL
Light oils, particularly good for the face. Use as part of a mixture.

AVOCADO
A rich oil, one of the most penetrative and easily absorbed. Particularly good for dry skin. Use as part of a mixture.

CARROT
Rich in Vitamin A. Also good for the face, but not always widely available. Only use in small amounts as part of a mixture.

JOJOBA
A form of vegetable wax. It is very rich and relatively expensive – best used on the face.

WHEATGERM
A rich oil, excellent for dry skin. It has a high vitamin E content, and is good for scar tissue and stretch marks. Use as part of a mixture, and as an antioxidant. Do not use if you have a wheat allergy.

Most vegetable oils, such as olive, may be used, but ensure the smell is not too strong.

ESSENTIAL OILS

BASIL (*top note*)
Basil is an antiseptic and nerve tonic. It is good for catarrh, sinus congestion, bronchitis, and indigestion. It has an uplifting effect, clearing the mind and relieving mental fatigue. Avoid during pregnancy.

BERGAMOT (*top note*)
Bergamot is an antiseptic, good for vaginal infections, cystitis, bronchitis, bad breath and sore throats. It is sedative and at the same time uplifting, helpful for anxiety and depression. (Do not use directly on the skin or when in direct sunlight.)

CAMOMILE (*middle note*)
Camomile is good for soothing inflammation, and is useful for ulcers, burns, diarrhea and migraines. It also relieves muscular aches. It can be used for painful or heavy periods, and on dry or sensitive skin. It is sedative and anti-depressant, calming the mind and nerves.

CLARY SAGE (*middle note*)
Clary sage is a nerve tonic and a sedative, especially good for nervous depression. It eases menstrual cramps and promotes labor. It is useful for inflamed skin conditions, and is mildly euphoric. Avoid during pregnancy. (Use sparingly.)

FRANKINCENSE (*base note*)
Frankincense is an astringent, and is useful for coughs, catarrh, cystitis and vaginal infections. It rejuvenates the skin, and has a soothing effect on the mind. It is safe to use during pregnancy.

GERANIUM (*base note*)

Geranium is a skin cleanser and tonic, as well as a mild diuretic. It is helpful for pains, burns, skin inflammation, diarrhea and ulcers, and can be used to provide hormonal balance during menopause. It sedates and uplifts, and is useful in anxiety states.

JASMINE (*base note*)

Jasmine is an anti-spasmodic, sedative and anti-depressant. It relieves menstrual cramps, promotes childbirth, is useful for coughs and catarrh, and can be used for dry skin conditions. It has a relaxing, uplifting, euphoric effect. Best avoided during first months of pregnancy.

JUNIPER (*middle note*)

Juniper is a nerve tonic, has a sedating effect, and is useful in states of stress and anxiety. It is a diuretic, blood purifier, skin tonic and mild astringent, and may be used for rheumatism, cystitis, indigestion, flatulence, eczema and oily skin. Avoid during pregnancy.

LAVENDER (*middle note*)

Lavender is one of the most useful oils of all. It is an antiseptic, relieves skin inflammation, and is excellent for burns and scalds (you can apply it directly on unbroken skin). It is also good for rheumatism, cystitis, and diarrhoea. It relieves nausea, headaches, vomiting, cramps and promotes childbirth. It is also good for muscular aches and pains. It is sedative and relaxing, relieving depression and nervous tension. If you only have one oil, this is the one to have.

MARJORAM (*middle note*)

Marjoram is a sedative and nerve tonic. A warming and comforting oil, it is useful for insomnia. It aids digestion, relieves muscle spasm and lowers blood pressure. It can be used for colds, headaches, constipation and painful periods. Avoid during pregnancy.

NEROLI (*base note*)

Neroli is sedative, anti-depressant and calming, excellent for insomnia, palpitations, anxiety and depression. It is also good for diarrhea. It regenerates the skin, and can be used on dry, irritated skin.

PATCHOULI (*base note*)

Patchouli is a stimulant and astringent. It aids mental clarity, can be used on irritated, cracked or aging skin, and is useful for water retention, diarrhea and constipation.

ROSE (*base note*)

Rose is an antiseptic. It is cleansing, soothing, promotes circulation, strengthens the digestive system, relieves constipation and normalizes menstrual flow. It is useful for mature, dry skin. As an anti-depressant, it can be used for nervous tension and stress relief, and is useful when suffering from grief.

ROSEMARY (*middle note*)

Rosemary is an antiseptic and stimulant, acts as a heart tonic, and relieves coughs and colds, headaches, stomach aches, palpitations, and diarrhea. It aids mental clarity and memory loss, and has a beneficial effect on the eyes. It acts as a cleanser, and is good for dandruff and toning the skin. It also relieves muscular aches and pains. Best avoided during pregnancy.

SANDALWOOD (*base note*)

Sandalwood stimulates the digestion, is useful for diarrhea, sore throats, catarrh and coughs. It is an antiseptic, effective in respiratory and urinary infections and excellent for relieving dry, inflamed skin. As a sedative, it can be used for nervous tension and anxiety.

YLANG-YLANG (*base note*)

Ylang-Ylang is a sedative and euphoric, and is used for anxiety and nervous tension. It lowers the blood pressure and is good for oily skin. (Use sparingly.)

USING OILS

Keep the base oils separate from the essential oils until you are ready to make up a mixture. To make up a bottle of oil, you will need about 50 ml of base oil. To this, add up to, but not more than, 25 drops of essential oil. This will be enough for six to eight massages. For a smaller quantity, halve the amounts. Kept in a dark, stoppered glass bottle in a cool place, the mixture should last between six to eight weeks. For one massage, you can use a couple of drops of essence added to a small bowl of oil.

Once you have chosen and mixed the oils it should be warmed before you massage, and applied by pouring a little onto your hands, never onto your partner's skin. (Note: Be careful around the eyes. Essential oils can sting.) Essential oils need to be pure. They are expensive because of the extraction process and the quantities needed to produce them – but they do last a long time.

For therapeutic purposes, always make sure you obtain the highest quality (absolute) of oils such as rose and jasmine. The advantage is they smell wonderful and you will only need small quantities, so the expense balances out. Essential oils can be used in other ways, in baths, as inhalations, or burned. A delightful addition to a massage is to scent the room with oils before you begin.

Recipes

Listed below are some recipes you might like to try out before experimenting with your own. All of the ingredients are readily available. Do remember that certain oils will tend to blend together better than others, and that when you are starting off, it is better to use them one at a time. The recipes are intended as an introductory guide only. In order to treat conditions, you should always seek professional advice.

Base Oils

BASE OIL
For 50 ml base oil:
Grapeseed oil 95%
Almond oil 5%
Half tsp wheatgerm oil (optional)

RICH BASE OIL
Grapeseed oil 95%
Avocado oil 5%
Half tsp wheatgerm oil (optional)

LUXURY BASE OIL
Almond oil 90%
Apricot or peach oil 10%
Half tsp wheatgerm oil (optional)

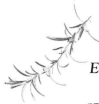

Essential oils to be diluted in 50ml base oil:

STIMULATING OIL
Lavender 15 drops
Rosemary 10 drops
This is good for relaxing the muscles
and clearing the system.

SOOTHING OIL
Camomile 15 drops
Lavender 10 drops
This helps nervous tension,
headaches and dry, flaky,
irritated skin.

WARMING, STIMULATING OIL
Rosemary 12 drops
Marjoram 8 drops
Basil 5 drops
This stimulates the system
and is good for colds.

UPLIFTING & REFRESHING OIL
Rosemary 12 drops
Bergamot 9 drops
Geranium 4 drops
This oil relieves nervous
tension and mental fatigue.

FRAGRANT, SOOTHING OIL
Rose Absolute 5 drops
Neroli 5 drops
Geranium 5 drops
This smells wonderful, is
calming and very good for stress.

RELAXING OIL
Lavender 12 drops
Geranium 8 drops
Sandalwood 5 drops
This is a sedating oil.

RELAXING OIL
Neroli 11 drops
Lavender 9 drops
Camomile 5 drops
Sedating, will help you sleep.

STIMULATING OIL
Rosemary 11 drops
Lavender 9 drops
Juniper 5 drops
This helps cleanse the system
and is good for cellulite.

SOOTHING OIL
Frankincense 16 drops
Rose Absolute 9 drops
This is great for the skin. (Note: Safe to
use after the fourth month of pregnancy.)

UPLIFTING OIL
Basil 11 drops
Jasmine Absolute 9 drops
This breaks the middle note
rule, but smells truly delightful!

HEADY, SOOTHING OIL
Lavender 14 drops
Frankincense 7 drops
Sandalwood 4 drops
This is an antiseptic oil, excellent
for the skin, and good for catarrh.

RICH, SOOTHING OIL
Lavender 9 drops
Frankincense 6 drops
Rose Absolute 6 drops
Patchouli 4 drops
This is luxurious, relaxing,
and good for mature, dry skin.

WARMING UP

Before massaging a partner, I recommend trying out some movements on your own body first, so that you can experiment with techniques and pressure, and feel free to make mistakes! On the following pages are some simple exercises through which you can explore the way your body moves and how the movements feel, plus a few warm-ups for your hands. Warming up before a massage is essential. The exciting thing about massage is that it is not only about using your hands, it involves using your energy as well. Follow the steps to stimulate the flow of energy through your fingers before the first massage contact. To put your partner at ease, have complete confidence in your touch.

RELAXED BREATHING
Main picture: Lie on your back, knees bent, and the lower back flat against the floor. Place both hands over your abdomen, and breathe naturally. Empty your mind, focusing simply on the rise and fall of your belly.

TURNING THE HEAD
Opposite top left: Sit in a comfortable position with your back straight. Turn your head slowly to the right as far as possible, and then to the left. Keep your shoulders still. Notice which muscles are involved in the movement, how far your head can comfortably turn, and any difference you feel afterwards.

FORWARD HEAD TILT
Opposite top center: Slowly tilt your head forward, chin toward your chest and back straight. Focus on the muscles. Feel how flexible they are, and at which point you feel a strain. Slowly raise your head up to the center again.

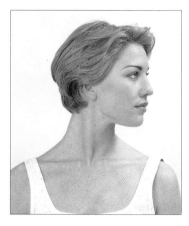

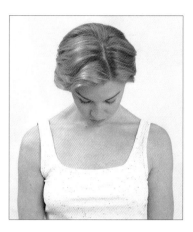

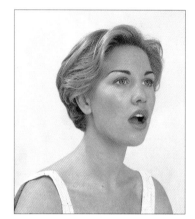

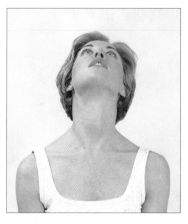

BACKWARD HEAD TILT
Right: Very slowly tilt your head right back, as far as feels comfortable. Keep your mouth and jaw relaxed so that your throat feels open. Feel the movement from inside, and notice any point at which you tense. Try doing this with your jaw tight, and feel the difference it makes.

RELAXING THE JAW
Above: Notice how you hold your jaw when your mouth is closed. Feel if the muscles are loose or clenched. Open your mouth, slowly dropping your jaw and consciously relaxing the muscles. Keep your mouth relaxed and notice if this feels new to you. Yawn if you want – it's a sign of letting go!

STRETCHING

Main picture: Either sitting or standing with a straight back, reach upward with one arm, stretching as far as you can. Then, stretch up with the other arm, each time reaching a little higher. Notice which muscles are doing the work.

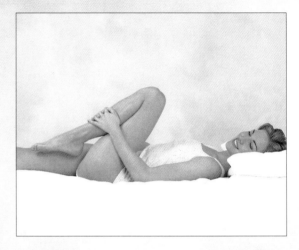

FLEXING THE HIP

Above: Lie comfortably on your back. Slowly bring your knee toward your chest, clasping your leg to help the stretch. Feel the muscles involved in the movement, breathe out, relax, and make the stretch a little tighter. Now do the same on the other leg, noting any difference in their flexibility.

FLEXING THE FOOT

Below: With one leg straight out in front of you, flex your foot, bringing the toes back toward you. Watch the muscles work, and really feel the stretch down the back of your leg. Breathe out, relax, and flex some more. Notice the feeling this leaves you with, and the way your muscles feel afterwards.

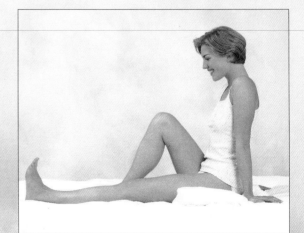

TENSING THE FOREARMS

Right: Holding your arms out in front of you, form your hands into fists, and tense the muscles as hard as you can. Feel how far the tension spreads, and the way in which your body is affected. Breathe out and release. Notice how your muscles feel immediately afterwards. Tense and release several times.

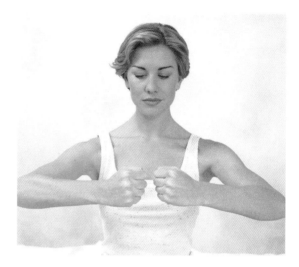

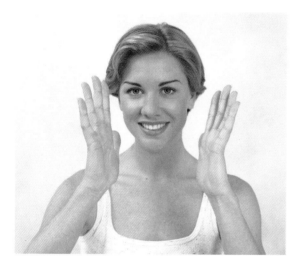

OPENING THE HANDS

Left: Make your hands into loose fists and hold them in this position for a moment. Then, quickly open your hands right out, stretching your thumbs and fingers as wide as you can. Repeat several times. Notice any different feelings in your hands. This is a good movement for flexibility.

FINGER WAVE

Right: Hold your hands in a relaxed position in front of you and then, leading with the little fingers, bring them all down, one after the other, toward the heels of your hands. Start again when the fingers reach the heel, so it is a continuous wave. This exercise is great for keeping the fingers light and flexible.

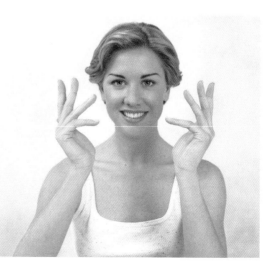

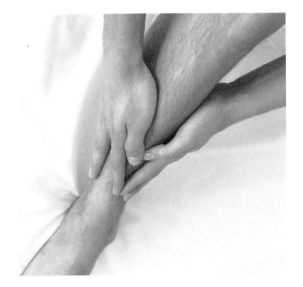

LEG EFFLEURAGE
Left: Sitting comfortably, reach forward and slide both hands together down the front of your leg, sliding right over the ankle. Reach around the back of the leg, bringing your hands up over the calf to the back of the knee. You can use more pressure on the upward stroke. This is a basic effleurage stroke.

TWISTING THE FINGERS
Right: Rest your hand in a relaxed position. Place the thumb and forefinger of the other hand at either side of the base of your finger. Twist the flesh away from you with forefinger and thumb. Twist up until you reach the tip of each finger, varying the pressure and speed.

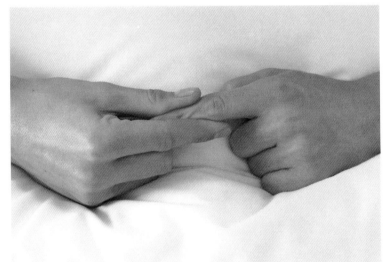

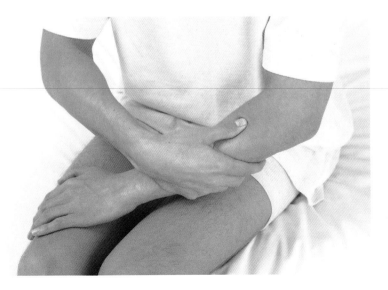

CIRCLING THE FOREARM
Left: Relax your forearm. Place your thumb in the center, roughly between the two forearm bones, and make small circling movements on the spot, using the pad of the thumb. Circle on the spot at intervals down toward the wrist, experimenting with different pressures.

PRESSING THE HAND

Right: Rest one hand palm upward and support it with your other hand. Place your thumb in the center of the palm, and simply press downward, then release. Continue pressing over the entire palm, trying out the movement at different speeds. Use the length, pad and tip of the thumb to vary the stroke.

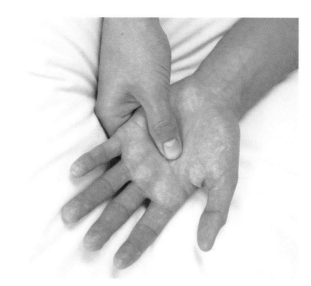

HACKING THE THIGH

Left: Raise your leg slightly and with your hands positioned sideways to the leg, chop down lightly on the thigh and then lift your hand up again. Hack with alternate hands, keeping your fingers relaxed and open. The movements, however, should be sharp and snappy. Hack quickly over the thigh.

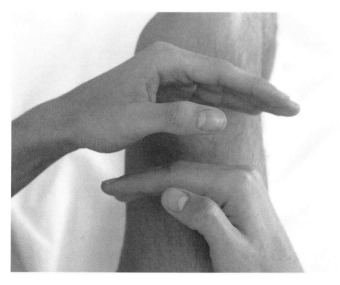

KNEADING THE THIGH

Right: Sit in a position that allows you to easily reach your thigh. With one hand grasp a roll of muscle, pressing in with your thumb and pushing it away from you. Then roll it back toward you with your fingers. Knead the thigh with alternate hands, finding the areas where the stroke is most effective.

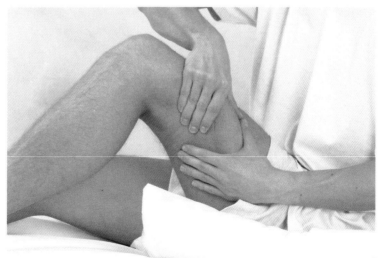

STIMULATING ENERGY
step 1
Right: Before massaging, you need to sensitize your hands and stimulate your energy. To practice this, sit or stand in a relaxed position, and begin rubbing your hands together vigorously. Feel the heat that is generated, particularly in the palms of your hands. Continue to rub for a few moments.

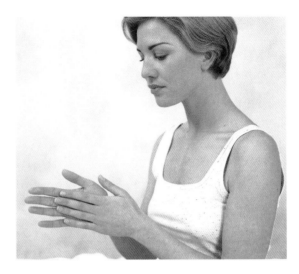

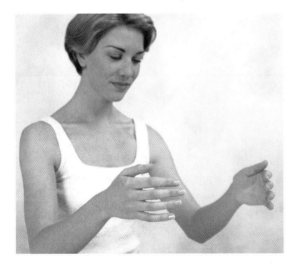

STIMULATING ENERGY
step 2
Left: Draw both hands apart to about shoulder width, and then slowly move them back toward each other again. When you are conscious of a sensation between the hands, stop for a moment, almost as if you are holding an invisible ball. Explore the sensation by moving your hands apart and together again.

STIMULATING ENERGY
step 3
Right: When massaging you need to feel, or imagine, that the energy is coming from the center of your body out toward your hands. Relax and breathe naturally. As you breathe out, feel the energy moving up from your abdomen through your body and then out through the palms of your hands.

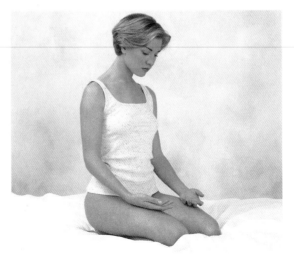

THE FIRST TOUCH

This will be your first contact in a massage sense, so the way you approach your partner is very important. Relax and breathe naturally, feeling the energy coming from your hands. Lean forward and place both hands flat on top of your partner's back. Just rest there for a moment. Your first touch and the feeling of your partner's back will speak volumes to you both.

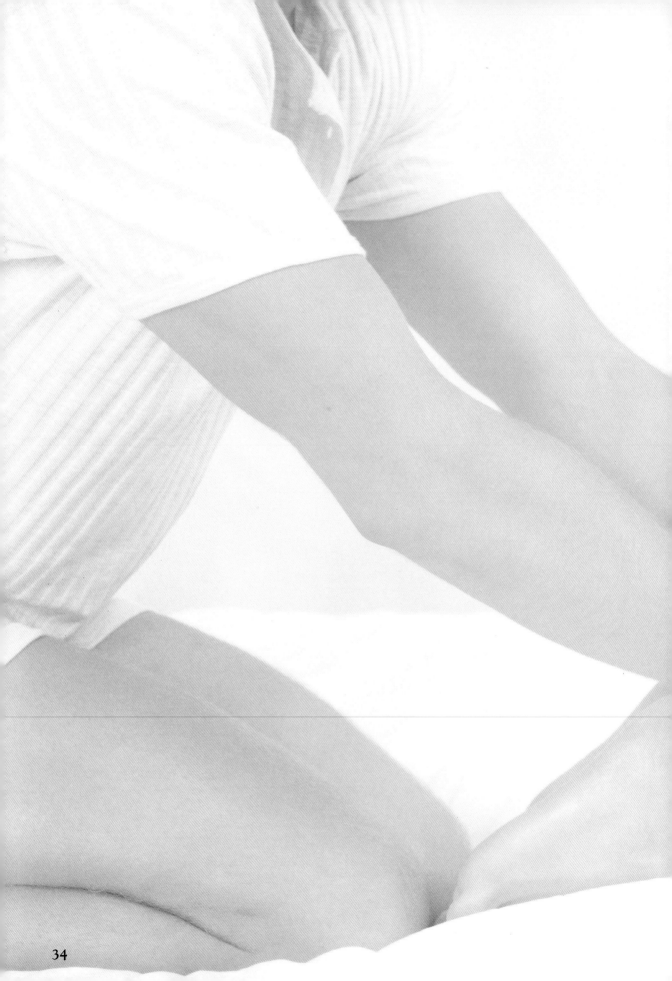

SIMPLE TECHNIQUES

The following techniques will provide you with the foundation for your first massage. These movements include effleurage, and kneading and squeezing – strokes which will always be included in any massage, as well as the softer, soothing strokes. Try out the techniques first as part of the massage preparation, becoming familiar with the parts of the body they are used on, as well as when they are used. As you practice, begin to get a feel for the amount of pressure needed. It will differ from person to person and depend on the area you are working on. Always make sure your own position is comfortable. You now have the essential ingredients for giving a massage at your fingertips.

EFFLEURAGE

Effleurage is the first massage stroke. It is used to spread oil over the body and to prepare your partner by relaxing the surface of the muscles. It also gives you a chance to "feel out" any areas of tension before you begin. Effleurage strokes are always very gentle, relaxing and reassuring. Effleurage each area with warm, oiled hands before massaging. (Never pour oil directly on the body.) Use large, sweeping strokes to cover the entire area, with greater pressure as you work toward the heart, and lighter on the downward stroke. Keep your hands relaxed, and mold them to the shape of your partner's muscles. Effleurage is soothing, and can always be used to fill in if you feel unsure of your strokes.

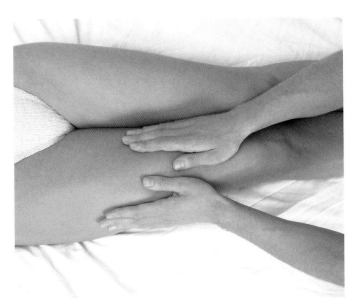

THE LEGS
Rub some oil onto your hands. Place the hands together over the ankle, then glide up the front of the calf, around the knee, and up over the front of the thigh. Separate your hands at the top of the thigh, reach up to the hip with the outer hand, and return down the outside of the leg, using a lighter pressure.

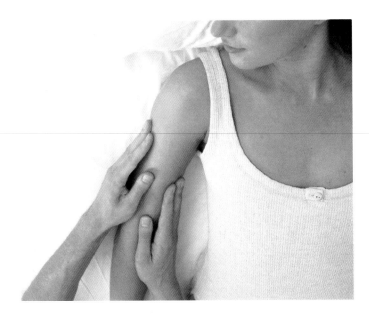

THE ARMS
Rub some oil over your hands. Place the fingertips together over the wrist, and slide up the center of the arm, reaching right up over the shoulder. Then, separate your hands, and draw them lightly down the outside of the arm returning to the wrist. Mold your hands closely to the shape of your partner's muscles and joints.

THE BACK

Oil your hands and position them together at the top of the back, fingertips pointing downward. Glide down over the muscles as far as you can reach, separating your hands over the lower back. Fan out to the side of the body, bringing your hands back up the sides of the ribs and around the shoulder blades to your original position. Stroke lightly off the neck or arms.

LOWER BACK & HIPS

Rub some oil onto your hands. Place them together in the center of the lower back, fingertips together. Circle upward, then spread your hands and fan outward over the hips. Slide around the hips and continue the circling motion back up over the buttocks. Return to the lower back, bringing your fingertips together once more.

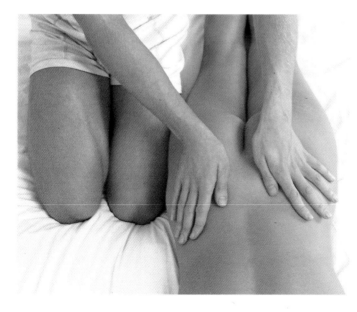

KNEADING

Kneading is a movement that really is a bit like kneading dough. It is done with the hands working alternately, squeezing and rolling the muscles. It is best used over soft, fleshy areas, like the buttocks and thighs, but can also be used over smaller areas, such as the shoulders or pectorals. The strokes can be done quite firmly, applying extra pressure with the thumbs, but avoid kneading directly over the bone. Make sure that the muscles you are working on are adequately oiled. Too little and you may pinch or pull the skin, too much and your hands will slide. Put your body weight behind the strokes, so the movements do not simply come from your hands. This is a deep, releasing movement used after strokes to prepare the muscles, and it will loosen and disperse tension effectively.

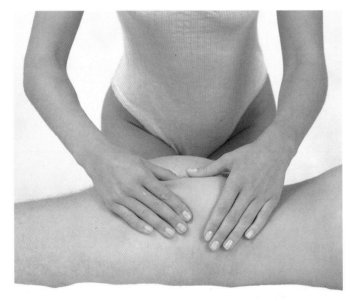

THE BUTTOCKS
You can knead quite firmly over this soft, muscular area. Lean over your partner. Press into the muscles with your thumb and push away from you as you do so. Then, roll the muscles back toward you with your fingers. Repeat the movement with the other hand, working in a gentle rhythm.

THE THIGHS
Place your hands over the muscles at the back of the thigh. Push away from you with your thumb, rolling the muscles back with your fingers, and continue the movement using your hands alternately. Knead over the thigh, but work only on the muscular areas, avoiding the inner thigh, knee and hip.

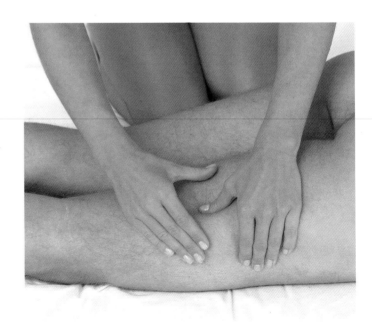

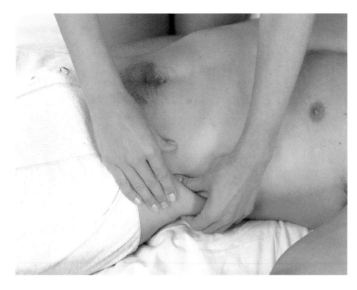

THE ABDOMEN

Left: Lean over your partner. Grasp a roll of flesh at the side of the abdomen, between the rib cage and hip. Press in with your thumb and roll with the fingers, alternating the movement with your other hand. Keep the strokes small. Be careful not to dig in too much, or work directly over the abdomen.

THE SHOULDERS

Right: Grasp the muscles that run along the top of the shoulder. Press in with your thumb, rolling back toward you with your fingertips. Knead along the shoulder to the neck and back. Again, your movements will have to be quite tight. Squeeze and roll the muscles firmly to ease and loosen any tension.

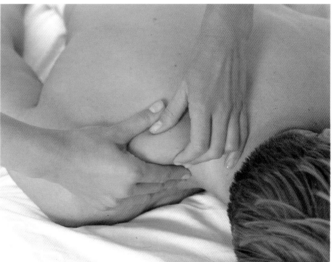

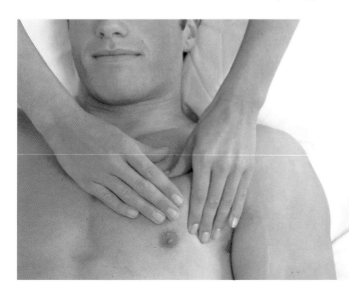

THE CHEST

Left: Place your hands over the pectoral muscles. Press in with the thumb and roll back with the fingers. Knead the area with your hands alternately, keeping your movements precise. Do not knead over the nipples, and for a woman, avoid the breasts. Squeeze and lift the muscles for extra release.

WRINGING

Wringing involves a pushing and pulling, twisting movement of the hands in opposite directions, which has the effect of pressing the muscles in between the hands as they move toward each other. It is used after kneading and squeezing strokes when the muscles have been loosened, and is often used to return the hands from one area of the body to another.

The strokes are as satisfying to perform as to receive. As the flesh twists, you can almost feel the tension being wrung and drained from the muscles. Wringing is used in a series of continuous movements on fleshy areas, where there is a good bulk of muscle to work with. However, with lighter pressure, it can be used over the arms as well.

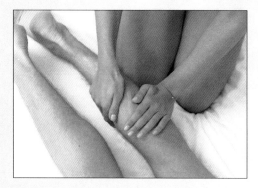

THE THIGHS
Right: Place both hands on either side of your partner's thigh, fingers pointing away from you. Push away from you with one hand, drawing back toward you with the other. Continue the movement as the hands cross, ending up again on opposite sides. Wring firmly over the thigh several times.

THE CALVES
Left: Place both hands over the back of the calf, one hand on the side nearest to you, the other on the far side. Push away from you with your near hand, at the same time pulling back toward you with the other. Twist the muscles as your hands cross, and continue the stroke up and down the calf.

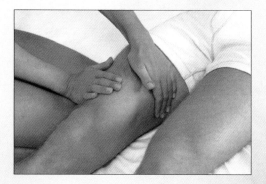

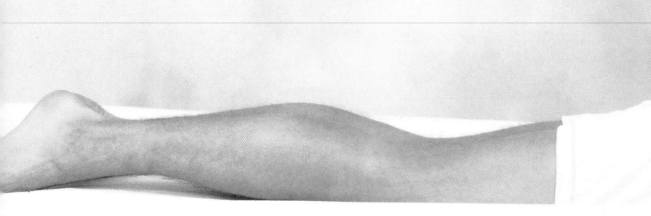

THE ARMS

Right: Place your hands on opposite sides of the upper arm. Push away with one hand while pulling back with the other. Continue the wringing movement all the way to the wrist, each movement leading into the next. Your strokes will easily cover the width of the arm and will need to be smaller at the wrist.

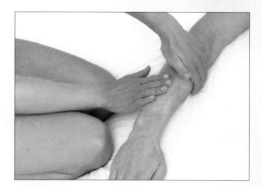

THE BACK

Main picture: Position your hands at either side of the lower back. Slide one hand over toward the center of the back, while pulling the other in the opposite direction. Use a firm pressure to twist the muscles in the middle. Continue the movement until your hands have reached opposite sides. Now, wring slightly further up and continue the movement up toward the shoulders and then back again.

PULLING

Pulling is a releasing stroke used to loosen up a whole area rather than a specific group of muscles, and is generally used after kneading. As you perform the stroke you pull against the body weight, so that it moves with your hands. The hands should be kept soft and rounded, beginning the strokes just beneath the body. As they slide up and over, so you release the muscles. Pulling is always done up the sides of the body, rolling the muscles as you work, and can be used to move from one area to another. You can pull the hands, one after the other, for example, at the abdomen, or travel along the body, hands crossing over as you move. Pulling can always be used when you are not sure of your next stroke.

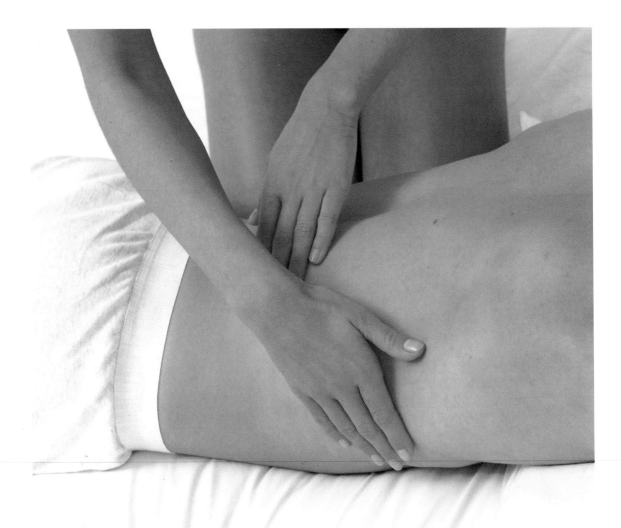

THE BACK
Lean across your partner, placing one hand under the body, just above the hip. Now, keeping close in to the body shape, pull your hand up and back toward you, lifting lightly off at the end. Follow this with your other hand slightly further up. Continue pulling, with hands crossing over, up the back.

THE RIBS

Lean forward, and place one hand just underneath the ribs. Pull your hand upward, and sweep around to the center of the chest. Follow this closely with your other hand, repeating the strokes several times. End by drawing the hands across the top of the chest and then stroking down the shoulder.

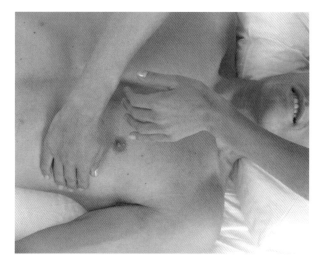

THE HIPS

Lean across your partner. Place one hand under the hip, and draw up and back toward you over the buttock, repeating the movement with your other hand. Pull with alternate hands several times. The body should rock with your strokes. Move up and down over the hips. End by lightly lifting your hands away.

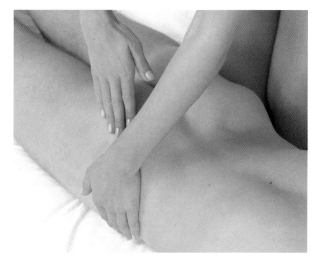

THE ABDOMEN

Lean over your partner and place one hand underneath the body, between the rib cage and hip. Pull back toward you, drawing your hand over the abdomen. Follow this with your other hand, repeating the movements several times. This feels particularly good the further under the body you are able to reach.

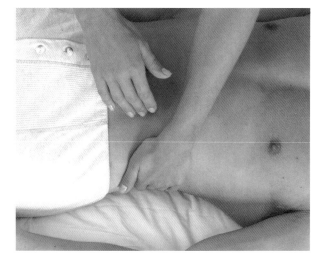

SQUEEZING

Generally the first stroke performed after effleurage, squeezing is done over the limbs using either two hands or one if the area is small enough. Squeezing movements are used across the shoulders, back and chest, although the strokes may take a different form to accommodate the shape of the body. The stroke is used to tightly squeeze the muscles, loosening tension in preparation for further releasing strokes. Squeezing the limbs is always done up the body toward the heart. Cover the entire length of the muscles in order the get the best results, always easing pressure as you approach the joints.

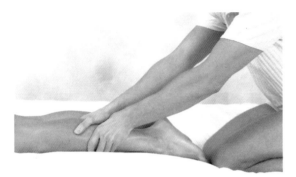

THE THIGHS
Right: Position your hands just above the knee, thumbs to one side of the thigh muscles, fingers to the other. Squeeze upward, spreading your hands as wide as possible. Push up to the top of the thigh, separate your hands, and round off over the hip. Repeat in strips up the thigh.

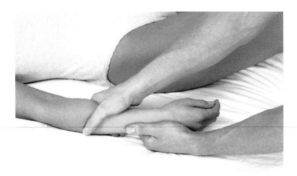

THE UPPER ARM
Right: Support the forearm and elbow. Position your other hand at the front of the arm, either side of the muscles above the elbow. Squeeze upward, pressing with your thumb, rolling the muscles between your thumb and forefinger. Work up the front of the arm several times.

THE CALVES
Left: Place both hands over the leg, just below the calf, with your thumbs to one side, fingers to the other. Squeeze into the muscles, forming a 'V' between your forefingers and thumbs. Squeeze up over the calf muscles, releasing the pressure as you near the knee.

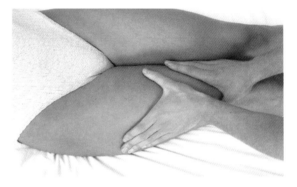

THE FOREARMS
Left: Support the arm at the wrist. Place your other hand over the forearm, thumb to the outside, fingers on the inside. Squeeze up the muscles toward the elbow, applying pressure between your forefinger and thumb. Repeat several times, easing the strokes at the elbow.

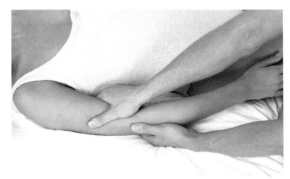

OPENING

Opening uses a spreading movement of the thumbs, or pressure with the heels of the hands where there is a larger muscle area. The strokes help to disperse tension after deeper releasing strokes. The opening movements move out across the body rather than up or down, although when performing a sequence you will generally stroke from the top of the body downward. Opening can return the hands to a particular position on the body, and can be interchanged with wringing. You then follow with softer strokes. Cup your hands right around the muscles to make the movements most effective.

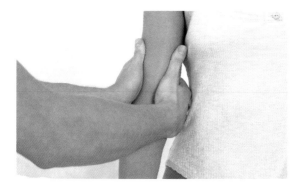

THE THIGHS
Right: Place both hands over the front of the thigh, thumbs together in the center, fingers cupped around the muscles. Press down and draw outward, using the heels of your hands to give firm pressure. Repeat the stroke up and down the thigh, easing pressure near the knee.

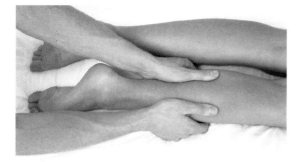

THE FOOT
Right: Place your thumbs together over the top of the foot just below the ankle, fingertips curled underneath. Slide the thumbs toward the sides of the foot, stimulating and squeezing the muscles. Use the pads of your thumbs. Repeat once further down, without pressing the toes.

THE ARMS
Left: Cup both hands around the upper arm and place your thumbs together in the center, facing you and pointing upward. Apply pressure and draw the thumbs outward to the sides of the arm. Repeat the movement slightly further down, and continue to the wrist.

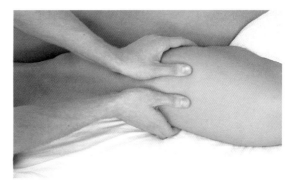

THE CALVES
Left: Cup your hands around the top of the calf, thumbs lying lengthways in the center. Draw the thumbs apart, spreading out across the muscles to the fingers. Work down the calf, releasing pressure at the bottom. Use the base of your thumbs to firmly squeeze the muscles.

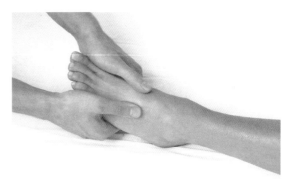

CIRCLING

Circling provides a soft, round movement over the body. The stroke can be used both for far-reaching release, as over the sacrum, or as a soothing, relaxing stroke, for example, over the abdomen. You can either circle with both hands, in alternate directions, singly, or with one hand placed on top of the other. Always keep your hands flat against the skin and very soft, even when you are circling over the bone. Circling can be used either to release or to gently diffuse the effects of kneading, and can often be used to replace pulling strokes up the body, or to return the attention, and your hands, from one area to another. It also gives a sense of movement and expansion, such as circling over the ribs, and brings a pleasant sense of softness to the body massage, and to your partner.

THE LOWER BACK
Right: Place one hand on top of the other over the sacrum (the bony triangle at the base of the spine). Circle the hands in an anti-clockwise direction over the sacrum and lower back, keeping the fingertips flat against the body. Keep your strokes precise, and avoid straying from the center of the back.

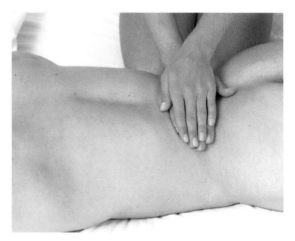

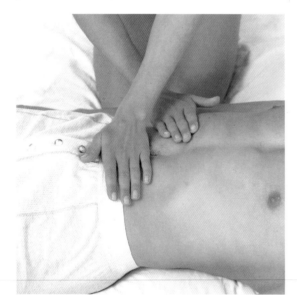

THE ABDOMEN
Left: Position both hands over the abdomen, one to either side of the navel. Slowly begin circling in a clockwise direction, hands flat against the body. As you circle, lift one hand to cross the other, so that you remain in continuous contact. Always circle gently, especially near the solar plexus.

THE BUTTOCKS
Right: Lean over your partner. Place one hand over the hip and circle in an anti-clockwise direction, then circle with the other hand the opposite way. Keep your hands flat and the movements firm. Make broad circles over the hips and buttocks, alternating your hands so that your strokes flow continuously.

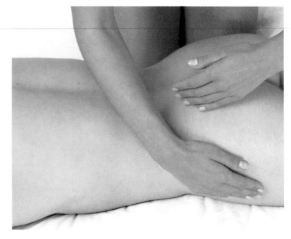

THE RIBS

Sit at your partner's head. Lean over as far as you can reach, and put your hands flat against either side of the body. Make big circles toward you with both hands at the same time, working up along the sides of the ribs. When you reach the shoulders, return to the bottom of the rib cage and repeat the circles twice, this time adding a slight stretch to the movements.

FEATHERING

In feathering you use the tips of the fingers to gently stroke down the body, alternating hands for a continuous rippling effect. It is one of the lightest, softest massage strokes, and one of the most delightful! Feathering is used to conclude after you have massaged each section of the body, or it can be used as a final stroke bringing the massage to a close.

Always stroke downward, and finally lift the hands so your movements will end almost imperceptibly. Feathering not only feels good, it serves a purpose, drawing the mind and senses down the body, connecting one area to another, and it can be used to draw tension out through the fingers or toes. Don't even feel tempted to skip it.

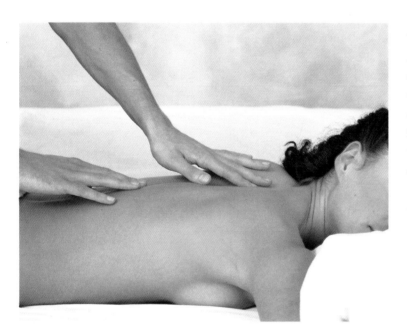

THE BACK
Left: Starting at the upper back, stroke very lightly downward over the skin with the tips of your fingers, lifting your hands lightly to begin the next stroke. Ripple down the spine to the lower back, then repeat the strokes twice more. Alternate your movements so that one hand is always in contact with the body.

THE ARMS
Right: Stroke with your fingers over the shoulder, and then continue to feather lightly down the arm to the wrist. Alternate the hands, starting the movements a little further down the arm each time. Lift the fingers at the end of each stroke, rather like stroking a cat. End by feathering the tips of the fingers.

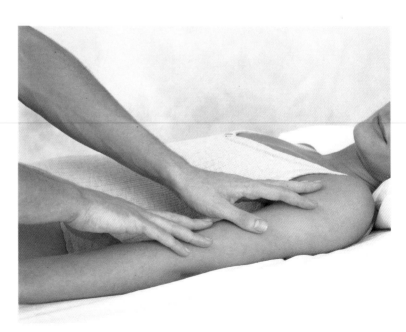

THE LEGS

Right: Begin this movement at the top of the thigh. Feather lightly down the leg and over the knee to the calf. Stroke with the fingertips, moving your hands alternately in a flowing rhythm. Stroke over the front of the ankle then slowly off over the toes. This gives the feeling of connecting the whole leg.

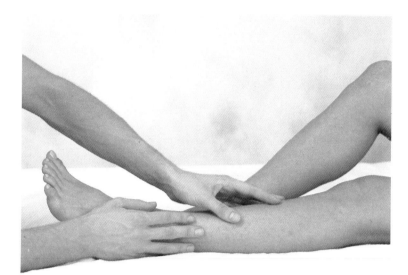

THE FEET

Left: Support the foot with one hand, and with the other feather in one movement from the heel to the toes. Repeat the soft stroking movements several times. Remember to stroke right over the tips of the toes, and to continue the movement for a few seconds after. Firmer strokes will prevent tickling.

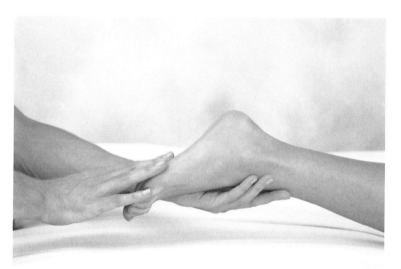

THE HANDS

Right: Hold the hand, palm upward, and with your other hand stroke lightly from the wrist to the fingertips. Draw your hand very slowly off the fingers, and as you do so, feel that you are drawing tension out through the body. These strokes can be very soft, following each other in waves.

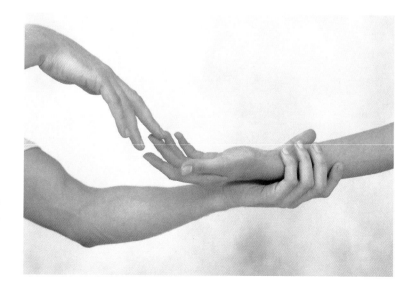

PRESSING

Pressing is a stroke performed with the pads of the thumbs. The thumbs can press alternately (as over the palms), singly, or one on top of the other (as over the forehead) where the body does not need to be supported. Pressing is used to release the muscles over a specific, usually small, area. The technique works best on soft, sensitive areas where you could not use kneading or squeezing, but are not too muscular so you can press over the bone. This type of thumb pressure aims at general tension release. You may cover pressure points, but this is not the main purpose of the strokes. The movements can either be slow and deep, or quicker to cover an area rapidly, and are usually used together with loosening strokes.

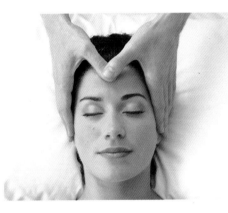

THE FOREHEAD
Resting your fingers at the side of the head, place one thumb over the other in the center of the forehead. Beginning just above the eyebrows, press lightly with the thumbs and then release. Keep pressing up the forehead, each time starting a little further up, and continue to the hairline, then repeat.

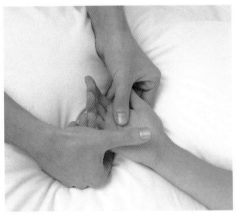

THE PALMS
Support the hand from underneath with your fingers, and place your thumbs over the top. Press down with the length of one thumb, release, and repeat the movement with the other. Press alternately with the thumbs quite firmly over the palm, with most of the pressure coming from the pads.

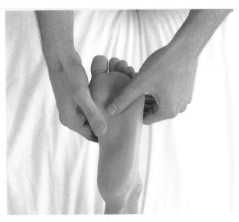

THE SOLES
Support the foot with your fingers, and place your thumbs over the sole. Press down with the length of one thumb, release, then press with the other, covering as much of the sole as you can. Include the heel, but be very gentle over the instep. Firm pressure avoids any accidental tickling.

RAKING

Raking is a wonderful stroke. By forming the hand into a claw-like shape, you then rake down or across the body, the hand shape allowing you to apply firm fingertip pressure. Unusually, the more angular your hands the better the movement works. Raking is rarely used on areas of the body other than the back, hips or tops of the thighs, where there is a lot of muscle. It is often used as the second half of a stroke, such as ironing or circling, over the spine and it releases tension down the back while at the same time returning the hands to the lower spine. Across the buttocks it can be used with pulling, after the deep releasing strokes. Be careful not to dig in too hard, and follow with soft feathering as a contrast.

THE UPPER BACK
Form one hand into a claw by raising the wrist and angling the fingers. Position it at the top of the back, fingers spread to the sides of the spine. Interlace your other hand so the fingers also touch the back. Pressing with the fingertips, draw downward over the muscles.

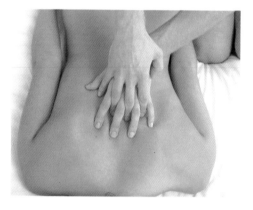

THE LOWER BACK
Spread one hand, fingers to the sides of the spine, in the middle of the back. Raise your wrists, form a claw shape, and press with the fingertips. Place your other hand a little further down, and, starting with the lower hand, draw both hands down to the lower back. Lift away from the body lightly.

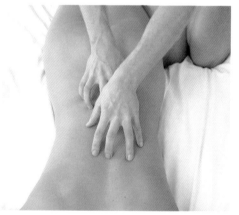

THE HIPS
Lean over your partner, and place one hand just below the hip. Raise the wrist and rake back up toward you over the buttock, and then begin the same movement with the other hand. Rake with the hands alternately. Continue the strokes over the buttock and hip, then rake over the top of the thigh.

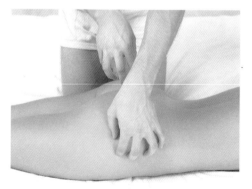

SIMPLE STRETCHING

Stretching is a beautiful addition to any body massage. Although working the muscles feels wonderful, the body can still feel compressed. Simple pulling or stretching affects the fibrous tissue around the joints and reduces muscle tension, leading to functional lengthening. Stretching gives a sense of expansion, taking the body beyond its functional limits and relaxing the muscles while restoring its range of movement. It should always be performed after the muscles have been warmed up and some of the tension released. The movements leading into each stretch need to be smooth, the muscles as relaxed as possible. Release the pull when you feel resistance and try again. Always stretch from a comfortable position.

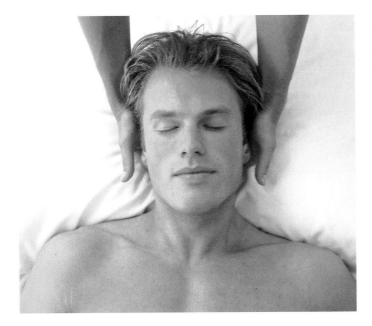

THE NECK
Place your fingertips pointing downward over the top of the chest. Draw over the shoulders and under the neck in one movement, cupping the hands under the base of the skull. Holding firmly, but without pinching, pull directly back toward you, then release, for a stretch down the spine.

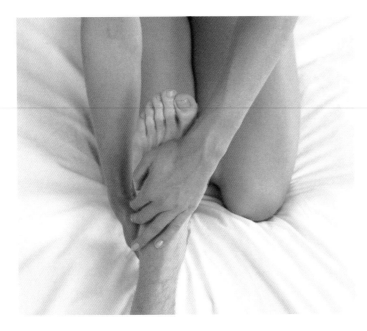

THE LEGS
Cup one hand under the heel of the foot, lifting the leg, and place the other hand over the top. Slowly pull back toward you, pulling mainly with the lower hand. Aim to get the movement coming from the hip. When you feel the joints resist, release and gently lower the leg, then try again.

THE ARMS

Grasp the arm at the wrist with one hand and lift it up, supporting it at the elbow with your other hand. Gently start to pull the arm upward, using your supporting hand to assist the stretch. Pull the arm up as high as it feels comfortable, and when you feel resistance, lower it back down folding at the elbow, then stretch up again. The pull should be able to be felt in the back.

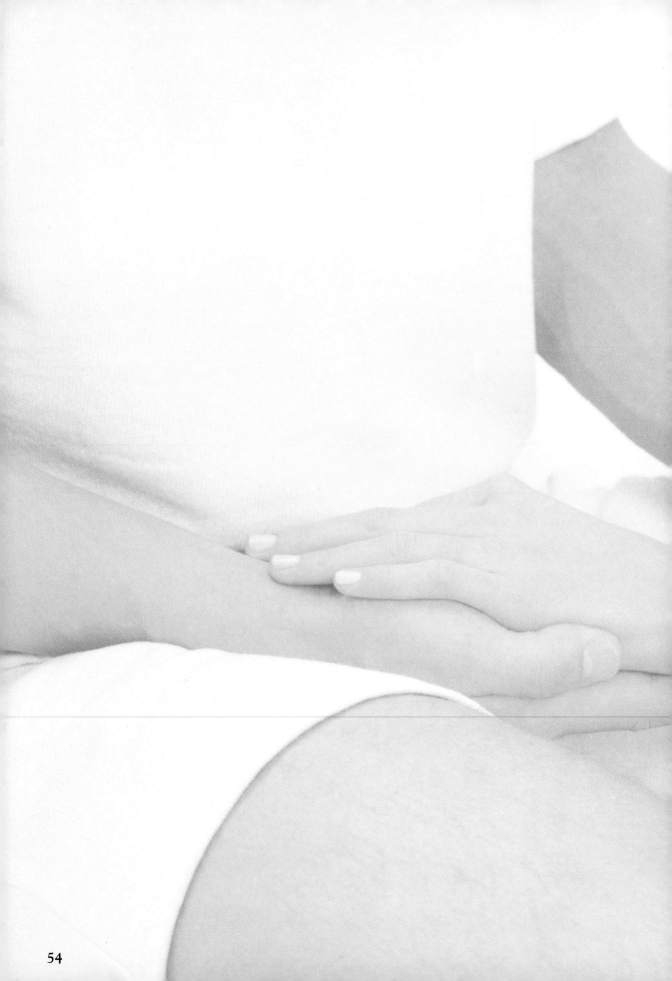

SIMPLE MASSAGE

The simple massage that follows is intended as a starting point, incorporating the techniques explained on the previous pages into a sequence that takes around 30 minutes. First master these simple movements, so that eventually you will be able to make up your own strokes and develop your own sequence and style. When you massage, always make sure you are in the correct position, with your back as straight as possible, and put your weight behind your strokes. While most people say they like firm pressure, err on the gentle side at first (you can always increase it) and check with your partner frequently. As long as you are sensitive to your partner's needs and health concerns beforehand, whatever you do is sure to be appreciated! The simple massage begins on the back, and leads to enormous rewards from your very first touch.

THE BACK

The back is the largest and most important area you will massage all at once and so the massage itself is divided into sections of the shoulders, lower back and spine. The back is a great opportunity to ease yourself into the massage, try out the techniques, and practice the long, sweeping strokes. Most people will feel comfortable about having their backs massaged, and are able to relax easily. Giving a back massage feels immediately satisfying because of the breadth of the muscles, and the fact you can actually see the difference you are making. As the back contains so many nerves and nerve endings, any massage you do here will have a direct and profound effect over your partner's entire body.

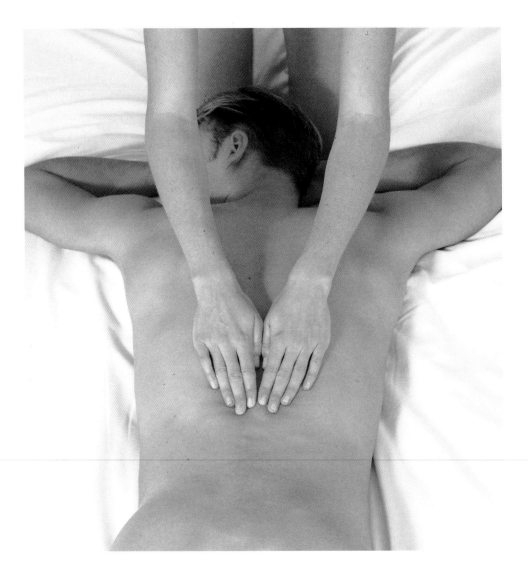

1. EFFLEURAGE *step 1*
Begin the massage by positioning yourself at your partner's head. Rub a small amount of warmed oil between your hands. Place both hands together at the top of your partner's back and start to glide your hands downward. Keep your hands relaxed and flat against the back, both spreading the oil and feeling out your partner's muscles.

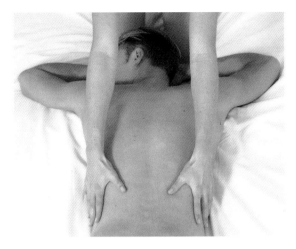

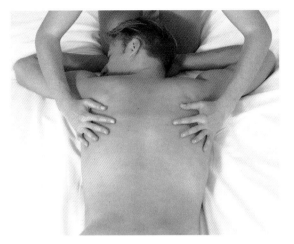

2. EFFLEURAGE *step 2*
Glide to the lower back, separate your hands and sweep out around the hips. Then, start to draw your hands back up the body, this time stroking up the sides. Raise your wrists, to increase the contact of your fingers with your partner's body. Reduce your pressure slightly on the return stroke.

3. EFFLEURAGE *step 3*
As you move right up the back, sweep your hands around the contours of your partner's shoulders, bringing your hands together again at the neck, and stroke lightly off the body. Repeat the whole stroke at least twice more, smoothing out your partner's muscles in preparation for the next stroke.

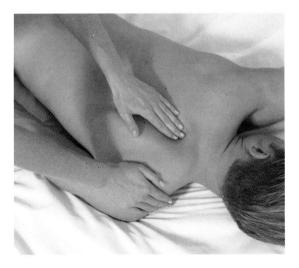

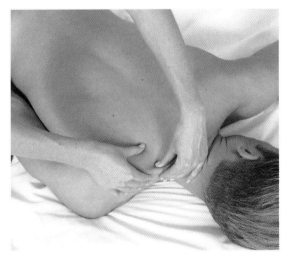

4. EASING THE SHOULDER
Move to your partner's side. Support the shoulder gently with one hand and with the other, press, circle and squeeze around your partner's shoulder blade, using either your fingertips or the flat of your hand. This is a loosening and relaxing stroke, easing and softening the muscles.

5. KNEADING THE SHOULDER
In the same position, begin to knead along the top of your partner's shoulder muscles, pushing in with your thumbs, and rolling your fingers back toward you. Continue massaging along the shoulder to the neck. As this is a fairly compact area, your movements will naturally be quite small.

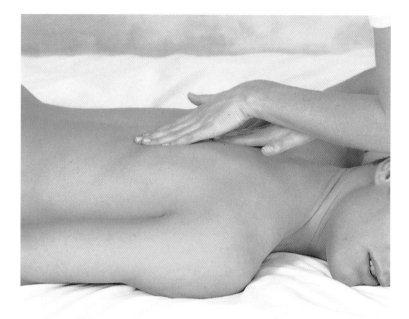

6. SHOULDER PUSH *step 1*
*Above: Return to your partner's head. Place the
fingertips of both hands, one behind the other,
at the inner edge of the shoulder blade. Now
push both hands slowly downward, pressing
firmly around the outline of the shoulder blade.
Follow the contours with your hands, at the
same time releasing any tension.*

7. SHOULDER PULL *step 2*
*Below: Continue the movement around the
bottom of the shoulder blade, then separate
your hands and draw them back up around the
rest of the blade, keeping close in to the armpit.
Your partner's shoulder should move as you
pull. Repeat the whole stroke. This is excellent
for loosening the shoulders.*

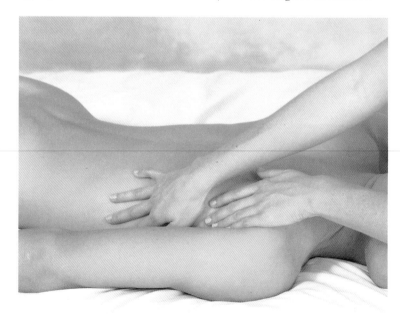

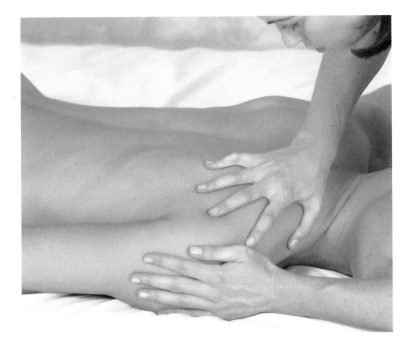

8. PUSHING THE SHOULDER DOWN
Above: After repeating the previous movement, end the sequence by placing both hands over your partner's shoulder and pushing the shoulder downward. The shoulder will move significantly, but only push as far as feels comfortable. Your partner will then feel a good release. Do the movement once only.

9. FEATHERING DOWN THE ARM
Below: Use the light feathering stroke to brush gently down your partner's arm with your fingertips. Use your hands alternately in a gentle rippling movement, as far as you can reach, in order to release tension down the arm. You are then ready to repeat the whole sequence on the other shoulder.

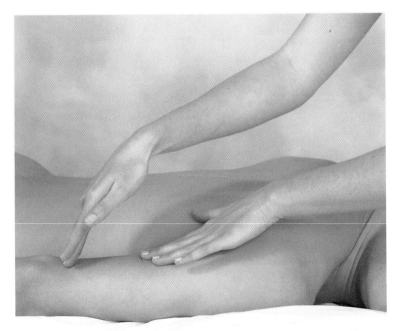

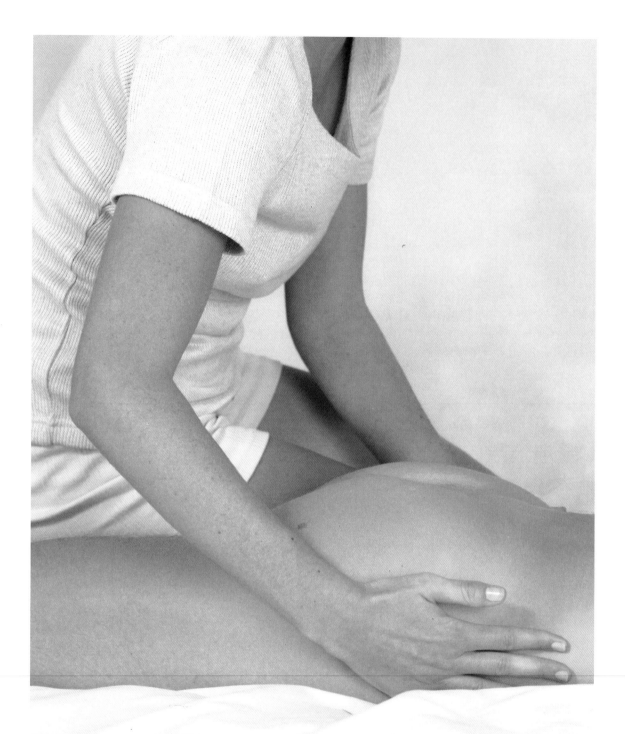

10. LOWER BACK EFFLEURAGE

Move further down your partner's body. Rub oil between your hands, then use effleurage strokes to spread the oil over the lower back, hips and buttocks. Start at the lower back, separate your hands out over the hips, come round the buttocks to complete the circle and return to the lower back.

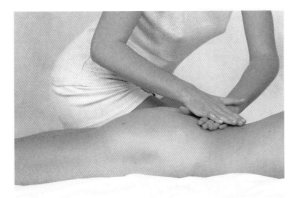

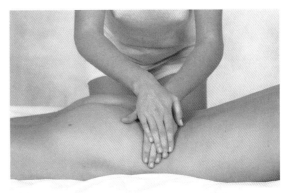

11. CIRCLING THE SACRUM
*Above: Place one hand on top of the other,
fingers flat, over your partner's sacrum (the
bony triangle at the base of the spine). Slowly
circle several times in an anti-clockwise
direction, using your upper hand for pressure.
This is a wonderful tension release, but always
check it feels comfortable for your partner.*

12. HIP PUSH *step 1*
*Above: Place both hands, one on top of the
other, in the center of your partner's back.
Start the stroke to the far side of the spine, just
above the level of the hip. Now, push away
from you, sliding your hands over the back and
downward, but keeping your stroke above your
partner's hips.*

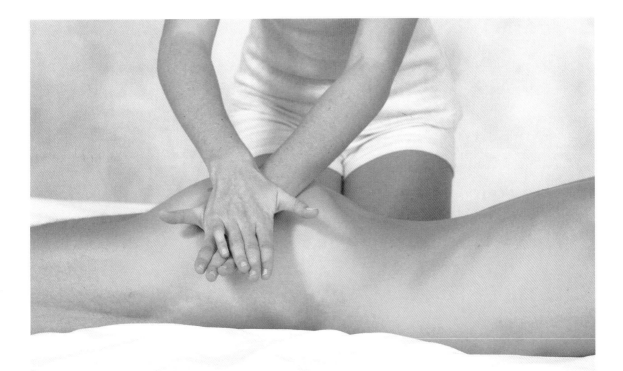

13. HIP PULL *step 2*
*Circle around the hip, pulling both hands back over your partner's buttock. As you pull, raise your
fingers so the pressure changes to the heel of your lower hand. Both steps of this movement flow into
each other, with greater pressure on the downward stroke. Repeat to release lower back tension.*

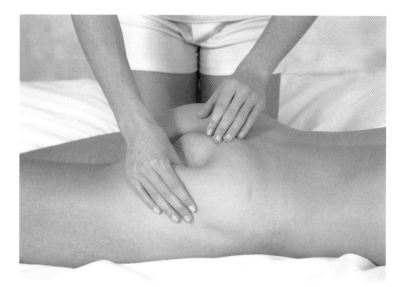

14. KNEADING

Lean over your partner, and begin kneading strokes on the buttock by pressing down into the flesh and away from you with your thumb, then rolling the muscles back toward you with your fingers. Move your hands in an alternating rhythm, and work only on the soft muscles, avoiding the bone.

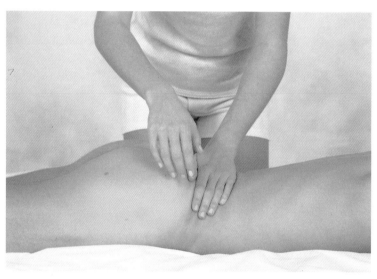

15. PULLING

Without breaking your movement, bring your hands just above your partner's hips. Slide one hand underneath the body, then bring your hand back toward you by pulling up your partner's side. Pull alternately with each hand, moving along the side of the body up toward the chest.

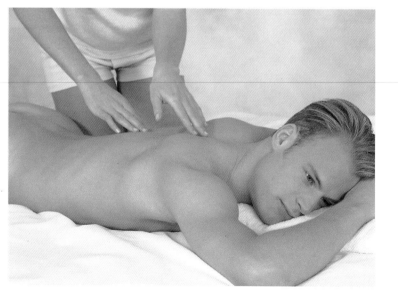

16. FEATHERING

When you reach the shoulder, use your fingertips alternately to softly feather the length of the back muscles, keeping to the far side of your partner's spine. Lift your hands away lightly at the end of each stroke. Repeat down the length of the spine several times, finishing at the lower back.

17. FOREARM STRETCH *step 1*
Lean across to the far side of your partner's spine and rest both forearms together, facing each other, in the middle of your partner's back. Keep your wrists relaxed and your hands formed into loose fists. Using your body weight, start to apply pressure downward with your forearms.

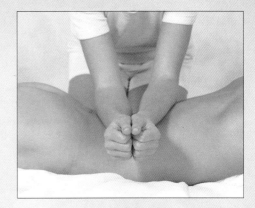

18. FOREARM STRETCH *step 2*
Main picture: Now turn your forearms over, and, still applying downward pressure, draw them slowly apart across your partner's back. Lean your weight into your arms and stretch until you reach the hip and shoulder. This not only feels great, but provides an excellent stretch for the muscles at the side of the spine. Repeat twice, change position, and perform the lower back sequences on the other side.

19. IRONING THE SPINE
Right: Place one hand on top of the other over the spine on your partner's lower back. Then, keeping your lower hand flat and using your upper hand for pressure, push lightly up the spine moving toward the neck. (This is one of the few times you will work directly on the spine itself.)

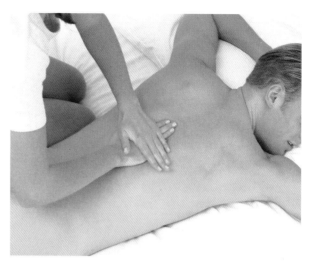

20. RAKING THE SPINE
At the neck, raise your wrists and fingers, and place one hand behind the other. Using the balls of your fingers rake down your partner's back, keeping your fingers to either side of the spine. Combined with the ironing movement, this is excellent for releasing tension along the spine.

21. STROKING THE SPINE

Return your hands to your partner's upper back, and stroke lightly down the spine several times. This is a profoundly relaxing and soothing stroke, which gives the feeling of connecting the entire back. It is also a stroke for warming down, and bringing the massage on the back toward its close.

22. RESTING

Right: This movement is deceptive, for it is not as passive as it appears. To complete the back massage, place both hands on your partner's back. Feel the energy coming out through the palms of your hands, at the same time feeling your partner's back coming into balance. After all the work you have done, it is important to spend a few quiet moments for everything to settle before you move on.

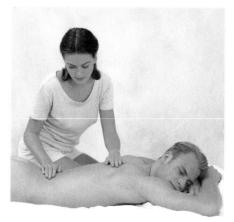

THE BACK OF THE LEGS

When you come to massage the legs you begin to feel a real sense of giving a full body massage. The legs offer you an opportunity to work on some of the body's most powerful muscles, and you can really get to grips with some of the basic strokes. While you should approach the legs as a whole, in reality your movements will be divided between the upper and lower legs, and the feet. The secret of a fantastic leg massage is to adjust your strokes to the length of the muscles, and not to taper off too soon. The leg stretch needs to be performed by you both confidently and comfortably, and gets better each time you practice. Once it becomes familiar, it will give the massage an added depth.

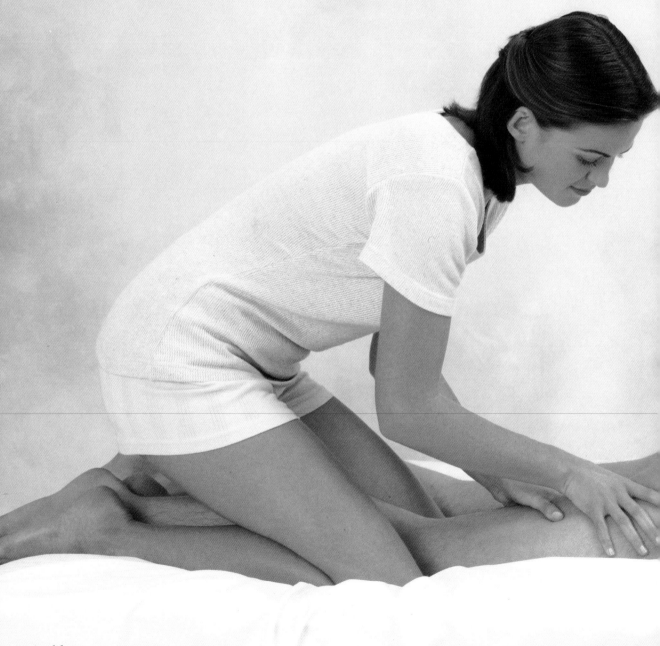

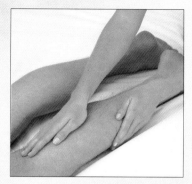
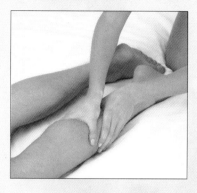
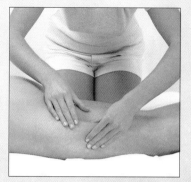

1. EFFLEURAGE
Position yourself at your partner's feet. Oil your hands, place them together above the ankle, and glide up the length of the leg, stroking lightly over the knee. Separate your hands, reach over the hip, and return down the outside of the leg. Repeat twice.

2. SQUEEZING THE CALF
Place both hands just above your partner's ankle, fingers and thumbs in a V-shape. Start to squeeze up over the calf muscles, spreading your hands as wide as possible. Release your pressure as you reach the knee. This stroke facilitates muscle drainage.

4. KNEADING THE THIGH
Change your position so you are square-on to your partner. Slowly start to knead the muscles over the back of the thigh. You can afford to use a firm pressure here, but check this as you are working. You will find the muscles move quite easily as you massage.

3. SQUEEZING THE THIGH
Main picture: Brush the back of the knee lightly, then resume the squeezing movement up the back and outer thigh, keeping pressure away from the inner thigh. Continue up to the hip, putting your full body weight behind the movement to achieve a good, firm pressure.

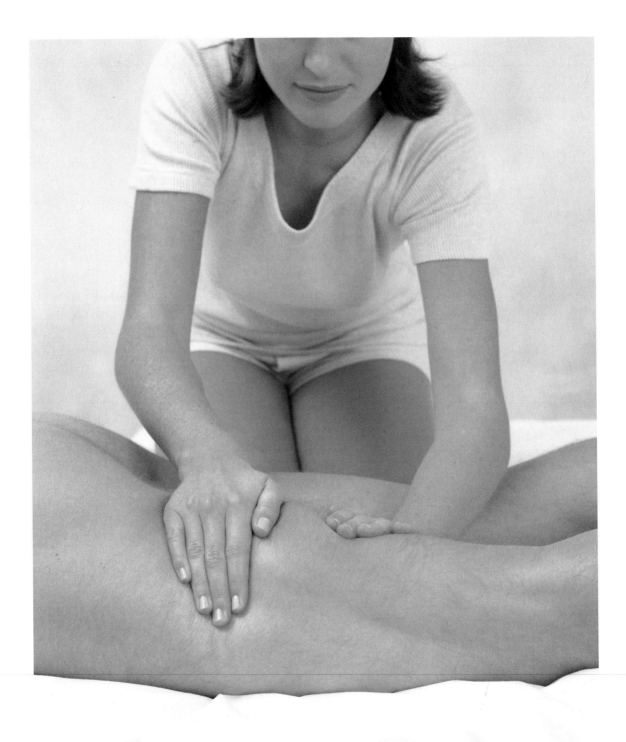

5. WRINGING THE THIGH

Place one hand over your partner's outer thigh, the other hand resting on the inside. Start to slide your hands toward each other, pressing the muscles firmly so they twist as your hands cross. Bring your hands to opposite sides of the thigh. Repeat the stroke the other way, working down to the knee.

6. STRETCHING THE LEG

Move to your partner's foot. Place one hand underneath the ankle for support, and your other hand around the heel. Now, use your body weight to lean backward, and pull the length of your partner's leg. You should be able to see this movement at the hip. The direction of the pull needs to be backward, rather than upward, and will give the leg a wonderful stretch.

7. PRESSING THE FOOT

Left: Gently lower the leg, and cup your hands around your partner's foot. With the balls of your thumbs, press right over the sole of the foot, covering it several times. You can use firm pressure, especially if your partner is ticklish, but avoid pressing over the instep.

8. FEATHERING THE LEG

Center: Use light feathering strokes which continue from your partner's hips right down to the feet. Move your hands alternately in long strokes down the leg. This gives a sense of connection, and brings attention to the feet. It is also a way of now bringing the leg massage to a close.

9. HOLDING THE FOOT

Right: Support your partner's foot from underneath with one hand, and lie the other across the sole, and simply rest for a moment. Focus on the energy coming from your hands. This will have a beneficial effect on the massage. Afterwards, repeat all the movements on the other leg.

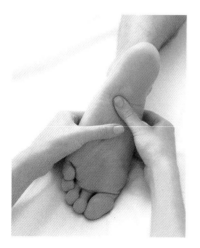
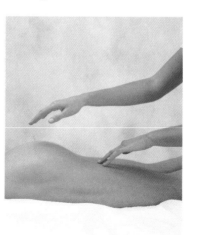
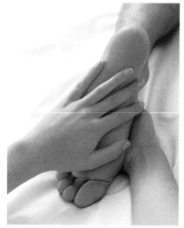

THE NECK

Front of the body massage begins at your partner's neck and is effectively a continuation of the back massage. In fact, the two areas should be seen as one, but it is easier and more effective to massage the neck in this position. As the neck can be particularly sensitive to touch, you will need to approach it carefully. Shown here are some simple but effective movements. The neck stretch feels absolutely wonderful and will make your partner feel at least two inches taller. Your partner should be encouraged to relax and simply let you do the strokes without tensing up or helping in any way. Try to keep your movements flowing and confident so your partner will let go and have total trust in your hands.

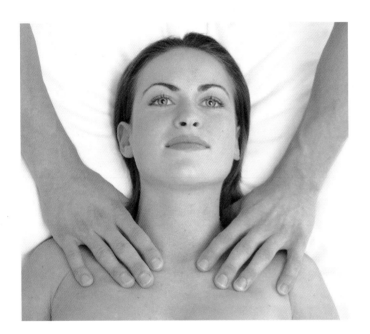

1. NECK STRETCH *step 1*
Left: Sit at your partner's head and rub a very little oil between your hands. Place them, fingers pointing downward, at the top of your partner's chest. Keeping your hands in full contact with your partner's body, draw them outward over the shoulders and slide round underneath the neck.

2. NECK STRETCH *step 2*
Right: Fingers facing upward beneath the neck, bring your hands back toward you until they are cupped around the base of your partner's skull and gently pull. The direction of the pull should be back toward you, rather than up. Only do this once. The two steps should feel like one movement.

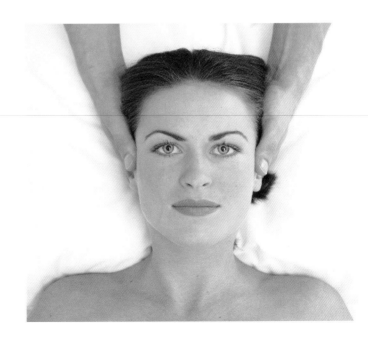

3. ROLLING THE NECK

Right: Now place both hands under your partner's neck. Start to draw one hand up the muscles at the side of the neck, rolling the head in the opposite direction. Then roll the neck the other way with your other hand, so the head turns back again. Roll the neck back and forth between your hands several times. Encourage your partner to relax during the strokes in order to feel the full benefit of the movements.

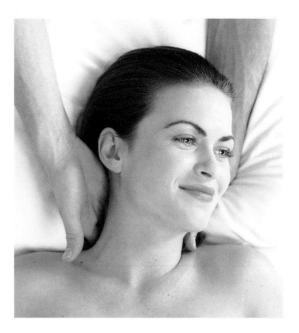

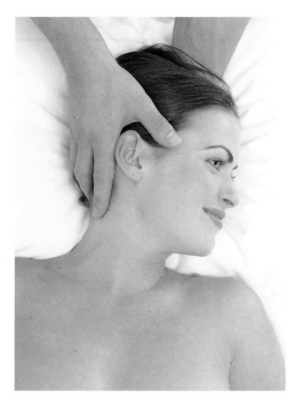

4. TURNING THE HEAD

Left: In order to perform the next movement, you will need to turn your partner's head. To do this smoothly, place both hands at the side of the head, thumbs in front of the ears, hands cupping the skull. Turn the head so that it rests on one hand, leaving your upper hand free to massage.

5. SHAMPOOING THE SCALP

Right: With the head resting on your lower hand, use your free hand to make shampooing movements over your partner's scalp. You can use quite firm pressure, as this usually feels fantastic. Cover the half of the scalp you can reach using the balls of your fingers, then turn the head to repeat the shampooing movements on the other side of your partner's scalp.

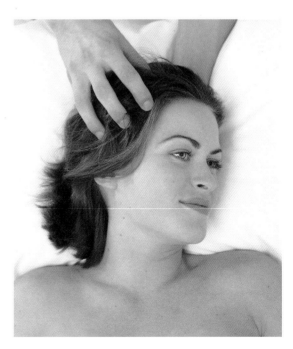

THE FACE

Having your face massaged feels blissful. A gentle face massage has a positive effect over the whole body and can really act as an aid to deep relaxation. Men and women alike can appreciate the sensation of the face muscles relaxing, particularly around the forehead and jaw. Keep your movements as delicate and precise as possible, making sure you don't lean any weight on your partner, and try to avoid accidentally brushing the eyes, eyelashes, or nostrils. Always be very sensitive. You can use either a very little, or no oil, but be careful not to stretch or pull the skin as you work. Make sure your movements always end in an upward direction, in order that your partner is left with a positive feeling.

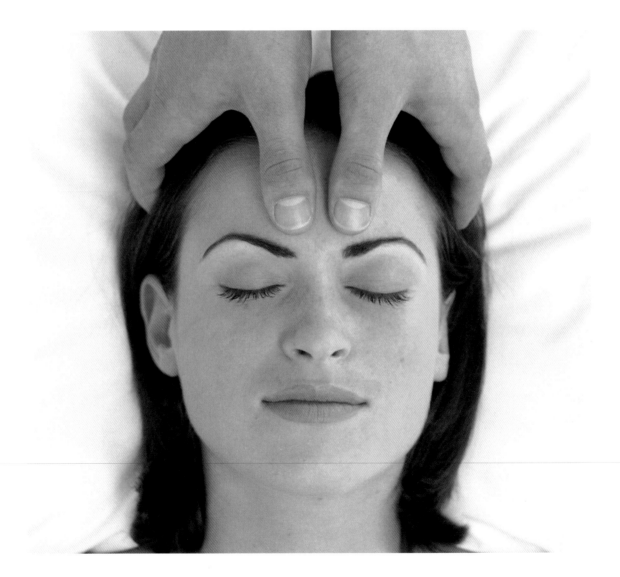

1. DRAWING ACROSS THE FOREHEAD
Cup your hands gently around your partner's head, without applying any pressure. Now place the length of your thumbs together in the center of the forehead, just above the eyebrows. Keeping your thumbs flat, slowly draw them apart until you reach the hairline. Have in mind the idea of dispersing any tension. Repeat this movement several times.

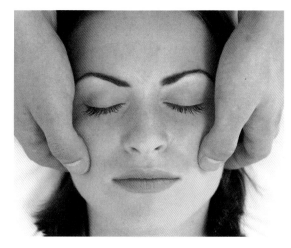

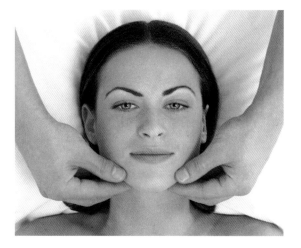

2. DRAWING UNDER THE CHEEKS
Resting your fingers at the side of your partner's face, place the balls of your thumbs beside the nostrils, just below the cheekbones. Once more, draw your thumbs apart following under the line of the cheekbones. Continue the movement toward the ears, ending with an upward stroke. Do this once.

3. DRAWING UNDER THE CHIN
Place your hands in the center of your partner's chin. Your thumbs should be just above the chin, your fingers just below. Now slide your hands out along the jaw line, squeezing gently between your thumbs and fingers. Follow round as far as you can, stroking upward toward the ears.

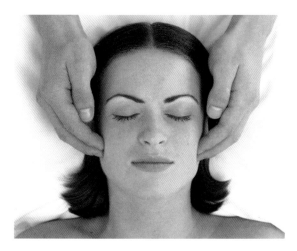

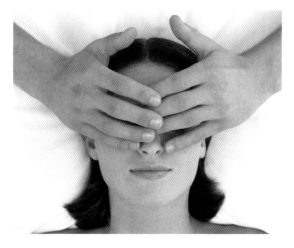

4. CIRCLING THE JAW
Place the pads of your fingers to either side of your partner's jaw, just below the cheekbones. (If you open and close your own mouth, you will feel the places where the muscles work.) Start to circle over the muscles very slowly for an effective release of tension. Make the circles quite large, keeping your fingers together.

5. RESTING
To complete the face massage, place your hands gently over, but not touching, your partner's eyes. Again, think of the energy coming through your hands. Hold your hands in this position for a few moments. As well as relaxing your partner, this movement both rests and revitalizes the eyes.

THE ARMS

The massage on the arms is similar in approach to the massage on the legs. While the arms should be regarded as a whole, you will find that your massage strokes naturally divide between your partner's upper arms, forearms and hands. The arm stretch provides an opportunity to work on the shoulder and back. As with the leg massage, the key to a successful arm massage is to follow all the muscles from beginning to end. Your partner should be encouraged to totally relax and not try to hold on or help. As the muscles are more difficult to reach with the arm lying flat, support it for most of the movements. The muscles may look delicate, but you will find that you can keep your pressure quite firm.

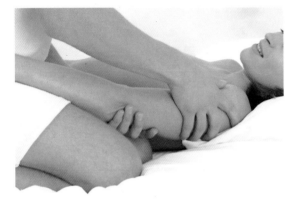

1. EFFLEURAGE
Move to your partner's side. Rub some oil onto your hands and then, beginning at the wrist, use effleurage strokes to spread the oil up over your partner's arm. Use greater pressure on the upward stroke, sweep over the shoulder, and return to the wrist. Repeat this stroke twice more.

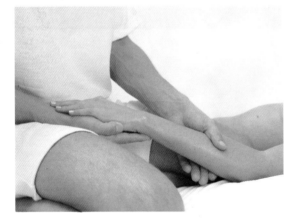

2. SQUEEZING THE FOREARM
Supporting your partner's arm with one hand, place the other over the forearm, thumb on top and fingers underneath. Beginning at the wrist, squeeze up along the length of the muscles, tapering off as you near the elbow. This stimulates the muscles and releases tension. Repeat this movement several times.

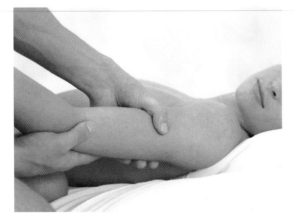

3. UPPER ARM SQUEEZING
Supporting your partner's upper arm, continue the squeezing movements between the thumb and the fingers. Start by beginning just above the elbow, and squeeze up the muscles to the top of the arm, reaching as far as you can. Apply most of your pressure to the front of the arm and repeat several times.

4. STRETCHING

Grasp your partner's arm at the wrist, and lightly support the elbow with your other hand. Pick up your partner's arm, and start to gently stretch it upward. Increase the stretch as far as the arm comfortably wants to go. As you pull, keep your support at the elbow, both to avoid any strain and to extend the stretch. Your partner will feel the movement in the middle of the back.

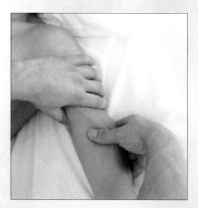

5. UPPER ARM KNEADING
Above: Lying your partner's arm flat, knead the muscles along the front of the arm. Push in with your thumbs and roll back with your fingers. Your movements will be quite small here. Knead up and down the arm several times.

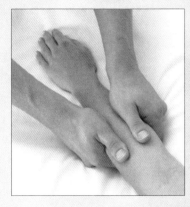

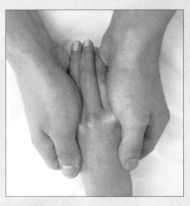

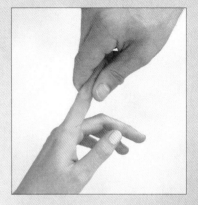

6. OPENING THE ARM
Place both hands around your partner's upper arm, thumbs together at the front, fingers cupped around the back. Slowly draw both thumbs apart, applying pressure with the base. Repeat the movement slightly further down the arm, and continue down the forearm to the wrist.

7. OPENING THE HAND
Place your hands in the same position over your partner's hand, and again draw the length of your thumbs apart. Keep your movement over the back of the hand, the pressure well above your partner's fingers. The hand will arch as you do this stroke, which has an excellent releasing effect.

8. TWISTING THE FINGERS
Put your thumb and forefinger around the base of your partner's finger and twist down the sides of the finger to the tip. You can do this stroke quite firmly. Twist down each finger of the hand in turn, including the thumb, loosening up the fingers as you do so.

9. PULLING THE FINGERS
Main picture: Hold one of your partner's fingers between your own, your forefinger over the base of the finger, thumb underneath. Slowly pull the length of the finger, coming off at the tip. Squeeze gently as you pull to draw out any tension. Repeat the movement on each finger in turn, then change your position to perform the entire sequence on the other arm.

THE CHEST

This massage affords you the opportunity to clear tension in the upper chest, the cause of which is particularly connected to the effects of stress. If you are massaging a woman keep your strokes either in the center of the chest between the breasts, or around the side of the ribs, but never massage the breasts directly. If you are at all nervous about this, keep your movements clear and confident, be very sure about the purpose of your strokes and then your partner will be able to relax as well. The shape of the ribs is great for strokes using the whole hand, and for molding your movements around the body. Pushing the shoulders reinforces the sense of lengthening and promotes total relaxation.

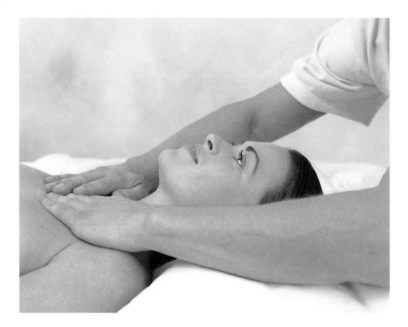

1. EFFLEURAGE
Move to your partner's head. Rub some oil between your hands and place them together at the top of your partner's chest. With your fingers pointing downward, glide your hands down the center of the chest to the bottom of the rib cage, using the tips and length of your fingers.

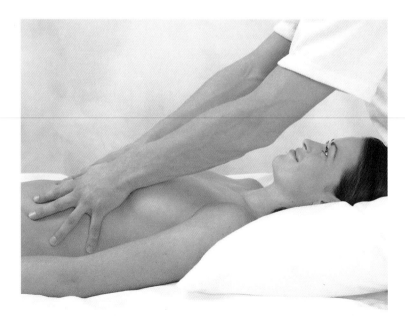

2. PULLING UP *step 1*
At the bottom of the ribs spread your hands, fingers pointing outward along the ribs, then draw them together and come back up the center of the chest to your starting position. Use lighter pressure on your return stroke, and finish using the tips of your fingers.

3. PULLING UP *step 2*
Repeat the effleurage stroke down the center of your partner's chest, but this time spread your hands right around the ribs, and pull up the sides of your partner's body. Keep your hands flat against the ribs, fingers spread, pulling very slightly as you return back to the top of the chest.

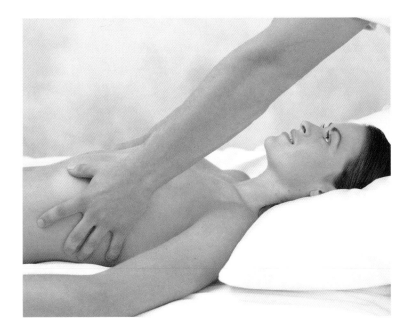

4. PUSHING DOWN THE SHOULDERS
As you return from the upward stroke, bring your hands to the top of your partner's shoulders. Placing both hands firmly over the shoulders, push downward using the palms of your hands. Push the shoulders gently down as far as feels comfortable, and you will be surprised how far they move. This will give your partner a great sensation of lengthening.

THE ABDOMEN

Massaging the abdomen is a special part of any body massage. We are all vulnerable and soft here, so whatever strokes you apply will penetrate deeply. The key is to be gentle and sensitive, and of all parts of the body massage, to think positively. Include the abdomen in any massage as relaxation here has a direct effect on the muscles. Over the abdomen you can use soft, circular movements using the flat of your hands. Move clockwise in order to follow the direction of the large intestine. The abdomen picks up stress quickly, so any soothing strokes will help. Be sensitive to your partner's menstrual cycle. It is fine to massage during menstruation, but check that she is not too sensitive to be touched.

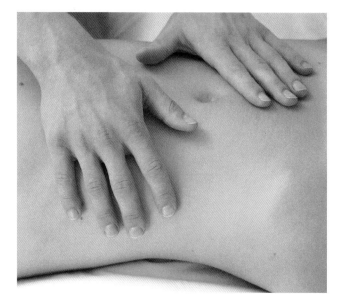

1. EFFLEURAGE
Left: Sit at your partner's side. Rub some oil between your hands, spreading it over your partner's abdomen using soft, slow effleurage strokes. Always make sure your hands move in a clockwise direction. Use the whole of the hands, keeping them flat, and ensure your movements are sensitive to help your partner relax.

2. CIRCLING *step 1*
Right: With one hand begin circling a little more firmly over the abdomen, still moving in a clockwise direction. Make your circle wide, taking in as large an area as possible within the boundary of the hips and rib cage. As one hand moves round, gently start to circle with your other hand.

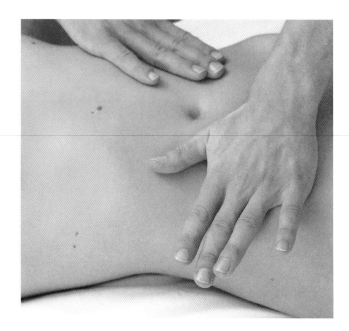

3. CIRCLING *step 2*
Right: As your hands continue the circle they will naturally cross over each other. Make sure you always keep one hand in continuous contact with the abdomen, and lift the other off as it crosses. This gives your partner a sense of continuity. Circle with soft, flat hands several times.

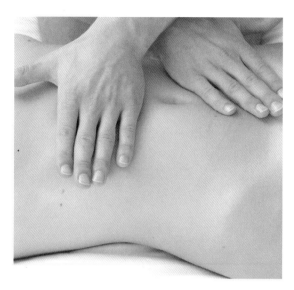

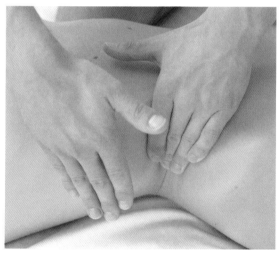

4. PULLING
Left: Leaning over, place one hand underneath your partner's body, just above the hip. Pull your hand back up your partner's side toward you. Pull with each hand alternately, using a reasonable pressure so the body moves as you do. Repeat this several times on both sides, changing position if necessary.

5. RESTING
Right: Place both hands flat over your partner's abdomen, and simply rest. As you do so, feel the energy coming out through your hands, and keep your thoughts positive. Make sure you do not lean any weight on your partner. This movement feels extremely powerful and will balance your partner's energy.

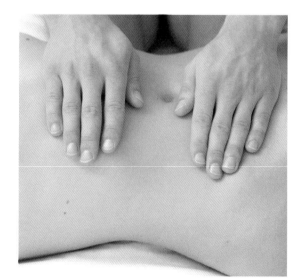

THE FRONT OF THE LEGS

This final part of the simple massage offers you an opportunity to work again on the legs and feet. You will now have covered all the accessible parts of your partner's body from head to toe. The fronts of the thighs contain powerful muscles, so even though you are bringing the massage to a close, your partner will miss out if you hurry. It is important to make sure your strokes cover the entire length of the legs, and especially go right over the hip. Every second you spend working the muscles thoroughly will be appreciated deeply, together with what is often sadness that the massage is ending! Make sure that you give time to the ending. It is as important as the way you begin.

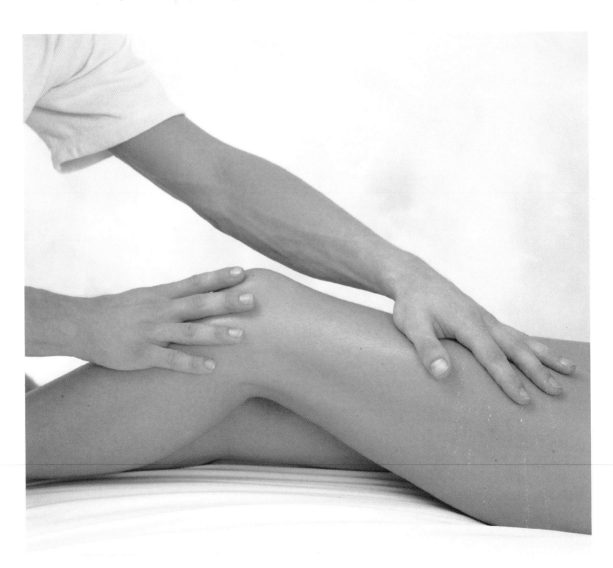

1. EFFLEURAGE *step 1*
Change position to sit at your partner's feet. Spread some oil over your hands and starting at the ankle, stroke up the center of the leg to the hip. You can apply gentle pressure on this upward stroke, making sure you reach right up over the hip with your outer hand.

2. EFFLEURAGE *step 2*
*Now bring your hands back down the outside
of your partner's leg to complete the effleurage
stroke. Keep your pressure light, and draw back
down the leg, raising your wrists so that you are
using your fingertips. When you reach the foot,
repeat the stroke twice more.*

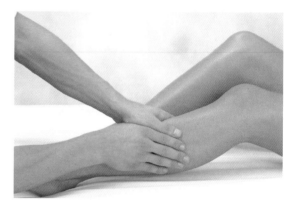

3. SQUEEZING THE CALF
*Place your hands over the front of your
partner's leg, just above the ankle. Have your
thumbs to one side, your fingers to the other.
Start to squeeze up the calf muscles, pressing
with your fingers and thumbs. Do not apply
direct pressure to the shin, and ease the
movement as you near the knee.*

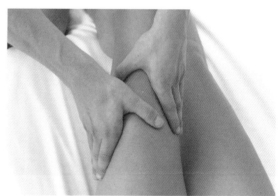

4. SQUEEZING THE THIGH
*Change position so that you can reach your
partner's thigh, and continue the squeezing
movements above the knee, your thumbs and
fingers on either side of the leg. Squeeze as far as
you can up the thigh, then round the movement
off over the hip. Repeat the stroke as often as
you need to.*

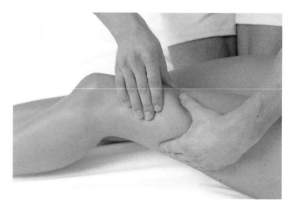

5. KNEADING THE THIGH
*Begin kneading over your partner's thigh,
feeling for any tension in the muscles and
working your way back down again until you
reach just above the knee. Work your way over
the front and outer thigh, keeping pressure
away from the inside thigh. Sit square-on to
your partner, and roll the muscles with your
fingers and thumbs, pressing the flesh in and
then rolling it back toward you.*

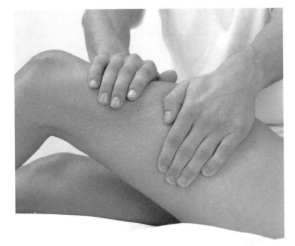

8. OPENING THE FOOT

Below: Cup your fingers underneath your partner's foot, placing the length of your thumbs together over the top. Draw your hands apart to the sides of the foot, pressing mainly with the base of your thumbs. You can do this movement several times, keeping your pressure above the toes.

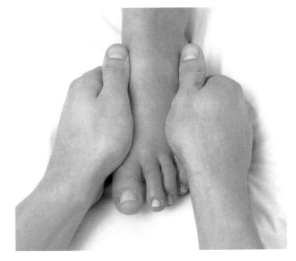

6. WRINGING THE THIGH

Above: Next, start wringing from the top of the thigh down your partner's leg. Placing both hands on opposite sides of the thigh, use a fairly firm pressure to bring your far hand back over the top of the leg toward you, your near hand pushing away from you. This produces a twist over the muscles.

7. STRETCHING THE LEG

Below: Move to your partner's feet. Place one hand underneath the heel and the other over the top of the foot. Lift the leg slightly, and pull slowly back toward you. This should be a comfortable stretch for your partner. The pull comes from your lower hand, your upper one is mainly supporting.

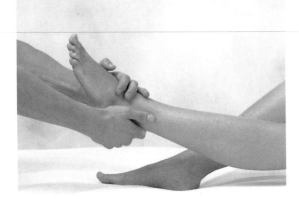

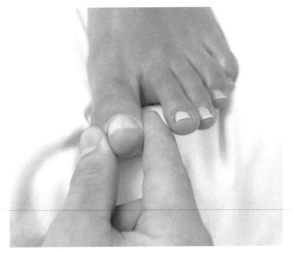

9. PULLING THE TOES

Above: Take hold of your partner's toe between your thumb and forefinger. Gently wriggle up the side of the toe toward you, pulling as you continue off at the end. Slowly pull each toe in turn, keeping your pressure firm if your partner is ticklish. This movement will feel truly delightful.

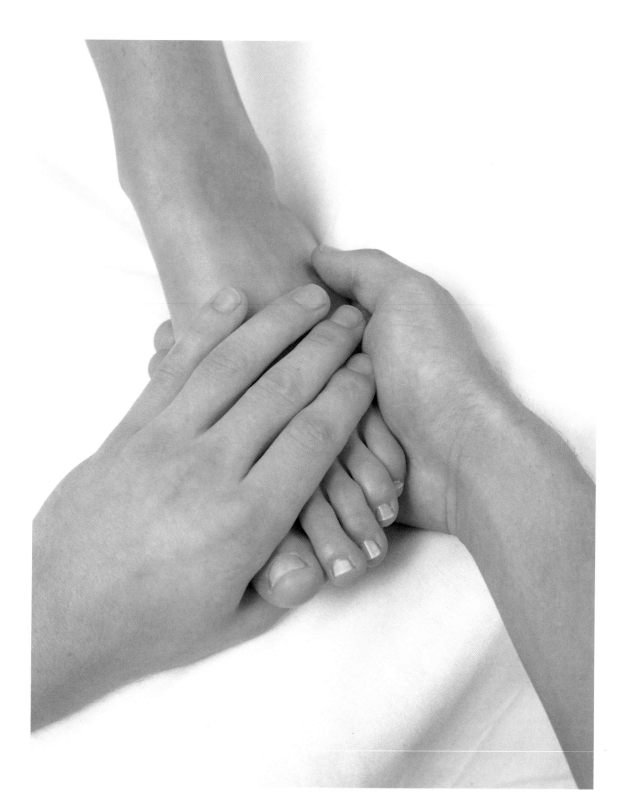

10. RESTING

Wrap your hands softly around your partner's foot, and just hold for a moment. Feel the energy coming through your hands. Make this ending soft but definite, before repeating the same sequence on the other leg.

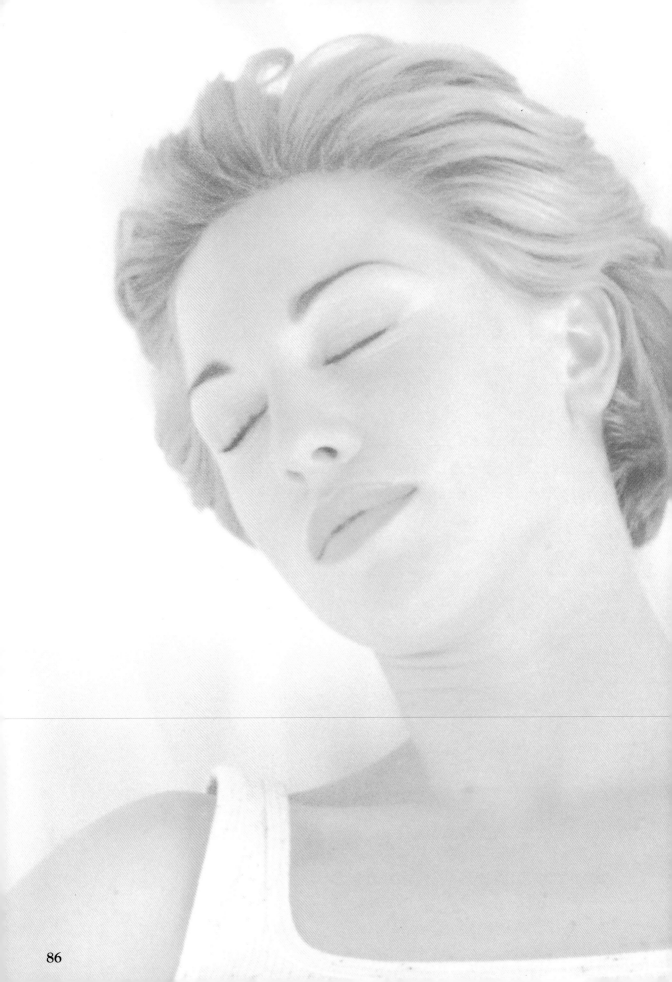

AFTER MASSAGE

Just as time and thought needs to be given to prepare for a massage, so too you need to give careful attention to the way your massage ends to leave a lasting impression. Some knowledge of what to expect is particularly useful when you are just starting. You can then make sure both of you make the most of it. The after-effects of a massage should never be under-estimated. For your partner, this means taking care to stay relaxed for at least an hour after, and for you, it means making sure you replenish your energy and give some time to yourself. Plan for this time in your general massage preparation, and be prepared for your friends to return for your services again and again!

THE AFTER-EFFECTS OF MASSAGE

Everyone reacts differently after a massage. The response is very personal, and has a lot to do with a person's mental or physical state beforehand. It is better not to go into a massage expecting a certain result, as this can be limiting and puts pressure on the person giving the massage. You can, however, expect that most people will feel much more relaxed. In addition, their bodies and personalities will be softer, their skin clearer, their color healthier and their eyes clearer and brighter. Some people even have their most creative thoughts during a massage. Feelings may range from feeling mildly light-headed to something resembling euphoria. If your massage has been stimulating, then your partner may well feel more alert and energized. Others feel an incredible sense of heaviness and tiredness, and want to go off and sleep. Some people work up a healthy appetite, others feel as if they have just been exercising, and may even feel a little sore. This is because massage takes the muscles beyond their present limit. Nearly everyone feels much looser physically, and problems such as a tense neck or shoulders, sore backs and headaches will feel much improved, if they have not completely disappeared altogether.

It is possible your partner may feel emotional either during or after the massage, which may result in tears. This is perfectly normal. During a massage you are emotionally open, and this may bring a release. However, it is simply part of the clearing process, and your partner will then feel much better. If your partner has little reaction, do not be disappointed or feel that your massage has not been effective. On many occasions, people have told me of amazing changes that have only taken place afterwards! As the person giving the massage, you too will be affected. Massage will make you feel more energized, more in love with life, it should make you glow!

Guidelines

Here are a few helpful guidelines you might follow after the massage finishes:

• Leave your partner to rest for a short while. When ready to get up, advise them to roll onto their side. This is easier on the spine.
• After a massage, your partner should relax for at least an hour and drink lots of mineral water to cleanse the body. It is always nice to have some to offer.
• It takes from 30 minutes onward for essential oils to be absorbed and they may remain in the bloodstream for up to eight hours. To obtain the full benefits, your partner should avoid showering immediately afterwards so that the oils can take effect. When ready it is better to take a warm, not a hot, bath.

It is worth remembering that during the massage you will have been working for almost an hour, with your partner simply lying flat, and that your strokes will have been producing a state of relaxation. The change in blood pressure helps account for the sense of dizziness some people feel on getting up. There can also be a physical reaction where the symptoms might actually feel worse for a period of a few hours afterwards. This will gradually clear, leaving them feeling very good. Again, all of this is quite normal – massage is more powerful than you might think! Your partner will probably sleep soundly the night of the massage, and the effects should last from two to three days after.

However your partner reacts, massage is an opportunity to make friends or bring you closer, and it is always nice to make an occasion of it. Setting aside an afternoon or an evening, not only for the massage, but for time to relax and talk afterwards, is always the best idea. You might then go for a walk, cook a meal or go out. Sharing the time together afterwards will turn your massage into a memorable experience.

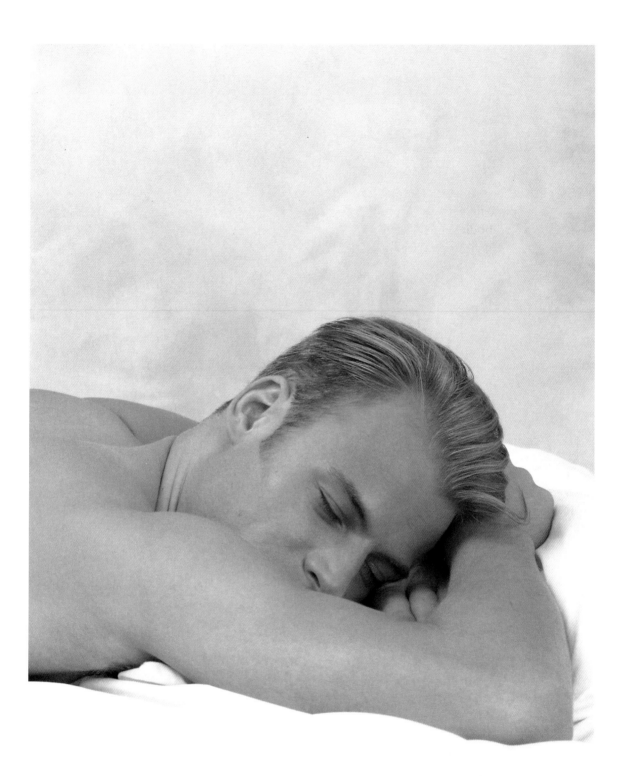

Feedback and reactions

Massage is a great time to get to know your partner better. Everyone reacts differently, has different needs and preferences, and each massage you do will be different from the rest. It is important to listen to your partner, to understand how they feel beforehand, and how they feel and react afterwards. You will learn a great deal from the feedback, and the more you massage the more you will learn and the greater your confidence. Be as receptive as you can while you are massaging, and encourage your partner at all times to tell you what feels good, what feels comfortable, and if there is anything that does not feel good or that they do not like. Always check your pressure frequently at the beginning. If your strokes are too soft and gentle, they will feel ineffective; on the other hand, massage should never hurt. There is a certain sort of pressure that feels as if it is doing good, but there is another which simply feels like pain, and this you want to avoid!

While keeping within your own capabilities, be prepared to experiment, and adjust the massage if necessary. If your partner simply wants to relax, be sure to set aside some time at the end to talk about how the massage felt, and how their body reacted. You can learn a great deal from the feedback your partner gives you, and any criticism should not be taken personally. It may simply reflect your partner's taste, and be nothing to do with your technique. At the same time, your partner will probably want to know what you have noticed, such as areas of tension, if he or she felt relaxed and so on. Your partner will also be able to learn a great deal from you. Any reactions from either side are helpful and useful, even negative feedback, and will only lead to an improvement. The best way is to regard the massage as very much a joint effort so get involved, and above all have fun, enjoy your massage and relax!

Adapting the massage

While keeping to your basic massage sequence, which is particularly important right at the beginning when you are just learning, it is important to be flexible and able to adapt the massage to your partner's needs. For example, if your partner is suffering from an injury, you would support the injury with a pillow and massage around but not over it. Similarly, if he or she cannot lie with the head to one side, place towels under the head or chest and have your partner lie with the hands supporting the forehead. Injuries, priorities, preference, sensitivity or lack of time may all mean that you need to adapt your massage to include certain areas of the body, and simply brush lightly over other areas.

It may be that your partner is particularly sensitive. Shyness, uncertainty and vulnerability may all mean that you need to approach gently and to carefully choose your strokes. This is something you will gradually pick up on over time. Sometimes as you touch you will reap more reward by holding back just that little bit in order to go a little bit further. To touch more deeply and effectively requires a sense of timing, sensitivity and detachment not always easy to find. As the person giving the massage, you should look on your partner in a non-judgmental way, and if this is difficult for you, it is something you will need to develop. At all times, however, you should make sure your strokes are clear and non-intrusive, as your partner should never be made to feel uncomfortable.

If your partner has to be active or work afterwards, then you will need to use the strokes in a slightly differently manner. Percussion movements and pressure points are particularly useful here, as they tend to have a more stimulating effect. Keep the general movements brisk and cup or hack over the back, for example, ending with light pummelling movements over the feet. Stretching and passive movements on the joints will also have the same effect, in preparing the body to be active. Bearing your partner's needs in mind through the massage will guide you, and your own alertness will have an effect on your partner's state of mind.

Warming down

One of the wonderful aspects of massage is that it is as good to give a massage as it is to receive one! Giving massage revitalizes your own energy, totally transforming your mood, making you feel more positive, giving a sense of balance, and providing enormous satisfaction. It is also great fun. In all the years I have been massaging, it never ceases to fascinate me. It is always different, often unpredictable, and has never yet been boring! It is also a way of looking after yourself. You will notice a lot about your own body and needs. However, it is tremendously important not to underestimate the fact that massage involves huge amounts of giving, and it can be physically tiring, or emotionally draining. This is particularly true at the very beginning when you are concentrating on so many things at once and trying to get everything right!

It is important to make sure you receive a massage just as often as you give one. In addition, if you follow a few simple ground rules and stick to them, however good you get, you will be able to avoid the pitfalls that so many people fall into.

• Always set a time limit for the massage, and keep a watch where you can see it. Be clear whether it is only you giving a massage, or whether you are doing a swap with your partner, and if so, when that will happen.
• Always wash your hands at the beginning and end of each massage. This is not only for obvious hygiene reasons and to remove the oil, it also has a psychological effect.

• Never massage when you are particularly tired or bad-tempered, as this will often prove more draining.
• Set aside some time to give to yourself afterwards, and allow a short period of rest. This can take whatever form you like, but the important thing is to take the time to recharge and put back what you have given out. Massage can be tiring, and involves you with your partner in ways you may not be used to. At the beginning, especially, it is very easy to overstretch yourself. Relaxing, some simple stretching, a good cup of tea, a rest, some music, a warm, relaxing bath with lavender oil or salt are all ways of warming down afterwards, making sure you gather and replenish your energy.

Conclusion

It is fairly easy to grasp the basics of the strokes and perform a massage that is pretty much technically correct. But how much more can be achieved when massage becomes an art, freeing up the tension formed from habitual body patterns and mental attitudes. Through massage you can tap into the spirit, creativity, spontaneity and naturalness which are so often buried under layers of routines, struggles and effort. Giving an inspired massage is like playing an instrument, as you watch the body respond, yield and soften, as tiredness and resistance give way to pleasure, harmony and balance. Massage is a transforming experience. It provides that sense of unity, connection and feeling of being whole. As you work on your partner, so your energy will increase, and as you join with the energy of your partner, so both of you will experience a degree of change. The fun starts when that added magical ingredient, which has nothing to do with the physical effects, takes over, and it is then that your strokes will become truly inspired!

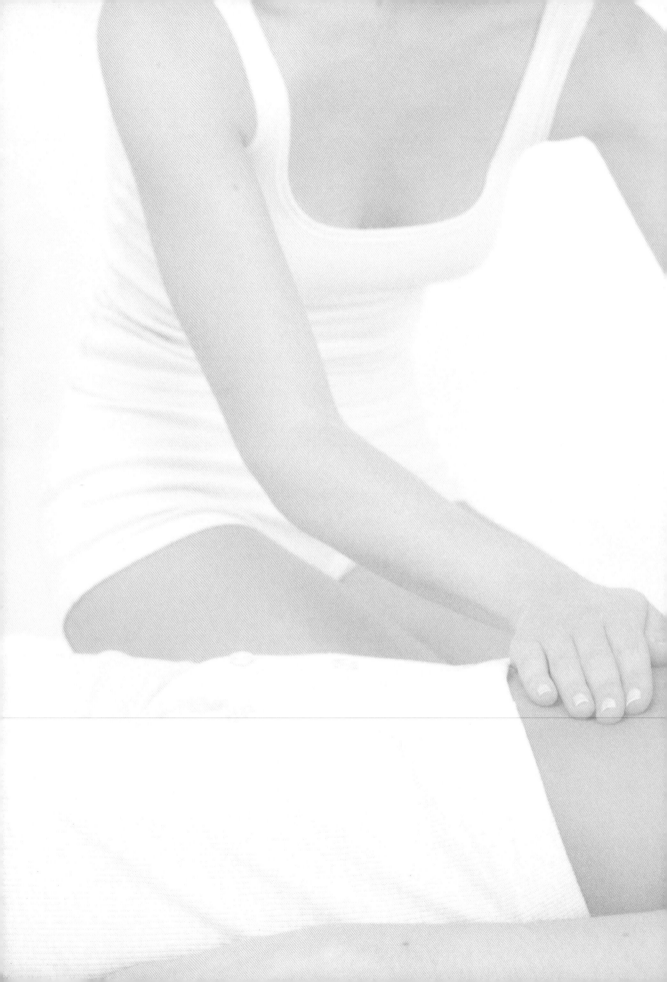

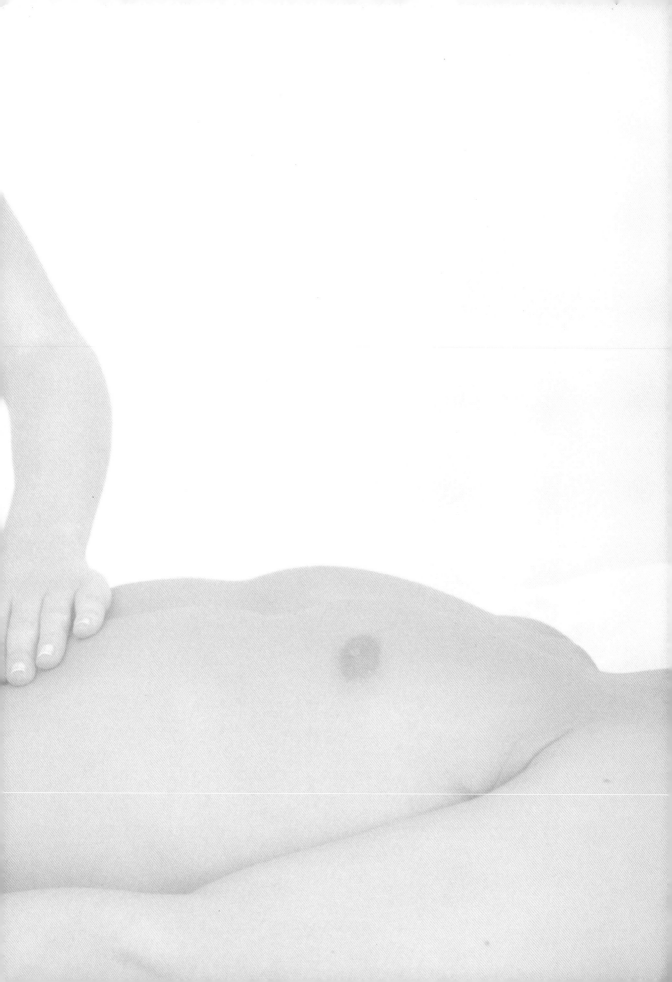

INDEX